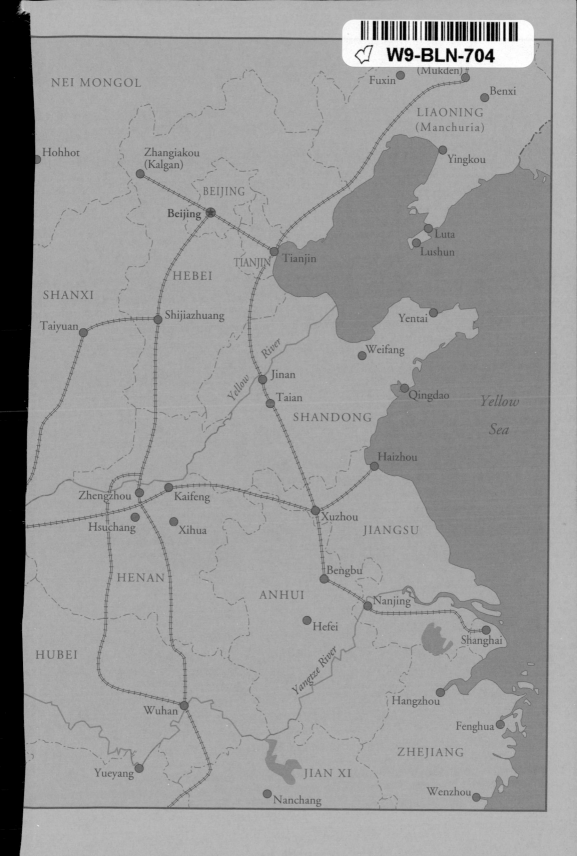

CHASING
THE
DRAGON

Also by Roy Rowan

The Four Days of Mayaguez (1975)

The Intuitive Manager (1986)

A Day in the Life of Italy (1989) Co-editor

Powerful People (1996)

First Dogs (1997)

Surfcaster's Quest (1999)

Solomon Starbucks Striper (2003)

CHASING
THE
DRAGON

*A Veteran Journalist's Firsthand Account
of the 1949 Chinese Revolution*

ROY ROWAN

THE LYONS PRESS
Guilford, Connecticut
An imprint of The Globe Pequot Press

Printed in the United States of America

ISBN 1-59228-218-0   •

3 5 7 9 10 8 6 4 2

The Library of Congress Cataloging-in-Publication Data is available on file.

For Helen,
who changed my life.

Contents

CHASING
THE
DRAGON

STEPPING STONES TO SHANGHAI

Lying awake in Shanghai's sweaty old Great Eastern Hotel, I was serenaded by the night sounds of the street below. It was more cacophony than symphony, although in time it was easy to identify the component noises as if they were coming from instruments in an unruly orchestra.

The clop-clop of bare feet on the pavement signaled a passing rickshaw. The rhythmic clack of chopsticks against a brass kettle revealed the presence of a noodle vendor summoning customers down to the sidewalk for a late-night snack, while the insistent cry, *"Membao! Membao!"* announced the arrival of a competing vendor offering steamed bread instead.

The pungent odor of their rival offerings blended with the stench of the "honey buckets" filled with human excrement, or "night soil," as it was called, being carted out of town to the surrounding farms for fertilizer. But it wasn't only the smell that informed everyone in the neighborhood of the honey bucket man's coming. His creaky old wheelbarrow, with its two iron-rimmed wheels, provided plenty of advance warning.

Screams, sirens, blaring radios, firecrackers, and tinkling pedicab bells added to the din echoing from Nanjing Road, the city's main thoroughfare. And the heavy clomp of shoes on the bare wood floor of the ancient hotel's hallway, mingled with the muffled patter of slippered feet, revealed the heavy traffic inside, as well.

That total assault on the senses was my introduction to China's teeming metropolis in July 1946. Sleep was out of the question. And, as it turned out, the hotel wasn't really intended for sleep. Only later did I learn that the Great Eastern, or "Greastern," as I called it in letters written to friends back home, was one of the city's flourishing brothels run by Du Yuesheng, boss of Shanghai's infamous Green Gang.

"Big Ears" Du, as he was known, had helped Generalissimo Chiang Kai-shek's Nationalists gain control of Shanghai back in 1927. When an early Communist cadre led by the young firebrand Zhou Enlai tried to take over the city, Du's thugs massacred most of the fleeing Reds. "Heads rolled in the gutter like ripe plums," according to one eyewitness. A number of Communist railway workers were also cooked alive in the boilers of their steam engines. Zhou, luckily, escaped. Dressed in a silk robe, fedora, and using a cane, the garb of a prosperous merchant, he boarded a ship bound for the Yangtze River city of Wuhan, known as Hankow when it was a cauldron of revolutionary zeal. "Big Ears" Du's reward for masterminding the massacre was the tight hold he still enjoyed on the city's variety of vices, from the opium dens in the old section of Nantao, to the waterfront bars of Hongkew, lined with smiling Chinese singsong girls and White Russian "hostesses."

Having arrived in Shanghai almost by accident, I wasn't prepared for such raucous surroundings, or for the city's clashing cultures. It wasn't just the stunning contrast of East and West or rich and poor that hit me so hard. I soon became accustomed to the procession of barefoot rickshaw boys padding down the street alongside sleek Rolls Royces, to the starving beggars sprawled on the pavement outside elegant restaurants, and to the marble banks and modern offices towering over ramshackle shanties along the Huangpu River esplanade called the Bund. Those sights were all too familiar in Shanghai. It was the inbred corruption and rampant violence that took some adjusting to.

Imagine a city that prided itself on having a street called Blood Alley. Or a place where an exasperated missionary once cried out, "If God lets Shanghai endure, He owes an apology to Sodom and Gomorrah." Yes, in the movies Marlene Dietrich had rasped, "It took more than one man to change my name to Shanghai Lily." And rollicking sea stories made it clear that this was where sailors really did get shanghaied. But I didn't expect the nonstop drama and excitement of this place, barely recovered from the "Dwarf Bandits," as the hated Japanese occupiers during World War II were called.

Shanghai, it soon became apparent, was actually several cities crammed into one. French Town accommodated Gallic transplants, who gathered in the afternoon for an aperitif and tennis at Le Cercle Sportif Française. The International Settlement was populated by Brits, whose favorite sport after a few pink gins followed by tiffin (lunch) was a game of lawn bowls on the manicured greensward of their Sporting Club. A few Yank businessmen tirelessly threw *Yahtzee* dice from a leather cup on the long mahogany bar at the American Club. An army of Austrian and Russian refugees rounded out the ranks of the resident *yangquizis,* as the local Chinese referred to all of us foreign devils.

In distant interior provinces the civil war between Mao Zedong's Communists and Chiang Kai-shek's Nationalists sputtered along, erupting here and there in quick-pitched battles, but with little sustained fighting. To the residents of Shanghai, that war in the summer of 1946 might as well have been taking place on another planet.

Yet it was because of China's civil war that I had come to Shanghai, after mustering out of the U.S. Army as a cocky twenty-six-year-old major. My last two years of the war had been spent in New Guinea and the Philippines. Perhaps it was the proximity of those Pacific islands to the Chinese mainland that lured me in the direction of Shanghai. But virtually all I knew about China came from reading Pearl Buck's *The Good Earth,* and from tales of intrigue recited by army buddies who had served in the China-Burma-India theater.

Hired by the newly formed United Nations Relief and Rehabilitation Administration (UNRRA) as a transportation specialist, my specific assignment had yet to be determined. The job description vaguely spoke of "facilitating the flow of relief supplies"—mainly food, clothing, and farm equipment—from Shanghai's port to the poverty-stricken villages of the interior. Be assured I wasn't a do-gooder out to save the starving Chinese. It was an innate desire for adventure and the hope of finding exciting stories to write about as a freelance journalist that lured me to China.

Ever since high school my secret dream was to become a foreign correspondent. That desire, as best as I can remember, surfaced in the ninth or tenth grade. My family was then living in Greenwich Village in New York City. The backyards of a dozen or so neighborhood buildings, most of them fronting on Bleecker Street, had been joined together to form a communal playground called Bleecker Gardens. Many of the residents were artists and writers. Renowned poet and English professor Mark Van Doren lived there. So did actor and playwright Franchot Tone and advertising copywriter-turned-novelist Jerry Carson. Our next-door neighbor was author/lawyer Roger Baldwin, founder of the American Civil Liberties Union.

Surrounded by such literary luminaries and given my own journalistic aspirations, it seemed only natural to start a newspaper, the *Bleecker Gardens Gazette* (I thrived on alliterations back then). This weekly had a staff of one. I wrote the articles, sold the advertising (fifty cents for a quarter page), mimeographed and stapled the pages, and delivered the paper door-to-door.

At Dartmouth College, my journalistic ambitions were further whetted by two stringerships—one as campus correspondent for the now-defunct *Boston Post,* the other for the *Springfield Republican.* The *Post* paid twenty-five cents an inch for every published story, the *Republican* fifteen. And since the two newspapers were miles apart and didn't object to running identical reports, the combined forty cents an inch came as a real bonanza.

My biggest college scoop came when Dartmouth's bruiser of a quarterback, Harry Gates, mysteriously vanished from the campus just a few days before the Harvard game. We finally tracked him down in a Vermont monastery. Harry had suddenly gotten religion, explaining also that he didn't want to play football anymore for fear of injuring an opponent. "Heavenly Gates," as he was instantly nicknamed in headlines flashed across the country, was finally coaxed back to the campus just in time for the game. If my ambition to be a reporter had ever wavered, this one colorful human-interest story that gained national attention clinched it.

While at college, I was also stricken with an insatiable appetite for adventure, a hunger that would eventually lead me all the way to China. It wasn't so much a matter of seeking thrills as a yearning for unique experiences to write about. This hunger for adventure led to jobs at sea during summer vacations. But they were hard to come by. It took several weeks of hanging around the Marine Firemen and Engineers Union hall to obtain a "trip ticket" for one voyage as a wiper on the tanker *Edward L. Shea*. Once aboard it was possible to keep making more trips until it was time to go back to school.

That tired old Tidewater Associated Oil Company tanker was spending its dying days plying between such unglamorous ports as Bayonne, New Jersey, and Beaumont, Texas. The destinations weren't very romantic. But for a wide-eyed college boy, the Texas ports provided a pretty good sex education. The bar girls in Beaumont, Port Arthur, and Galveston were not nearly as pretty as the ones I would discover six years later in Shanghai. But they were even more aggressive, grabbing at your groin and wallet simultaneously.

At sea, our tanker's shuttle runs were not the kind of voyages that inspired Joseph Conrad, one of my favorite writers. They were so monotonous, and with such brief periods spent in port, that it took extra pay and extra good food to keep the crew from jumping ship. However, the ocean's lonely beauty and limitless horizons always stirred my imagination.

I liked to stand on the forecastle head at night and peer down at a school of porpoises frolicking in the phosphorescent bow wake. Or lean against the stern rail under a sky full of stars and feel the whole ship shudder as the propeller churned out a frothy white path in the sea behind. During my free hours, when not standing a watch down in the engine room, I would try to find words to capture those inspiring moments.

Other times I would sketch the sea scenes in pen and ink. At Dartmouth, Paul Sample, the college's illustrious artist-in-residence had encouraged me to study with him, even suggesting that painting might be a more fulfilling career than reporting. But trying to make a living as an artist seemed even riskier in a grim economy still recovering from the Great Depression.

During my second summer at sea the union put me on a freighter named the *Floridian,* an American Hawaii Line rust-pot running intercoastal between Portland, Maine, and Portland, Oregon. Entering the Panama Canal on July 4, 1941, we encountered a small fleet of Japanese cargo vessels twirling idly on their anchor chains. The "Fuckyou Marus," as our crew referred to all Japanese freighters, had been banned from using the canal as of that date. The ban followed economic sanctions imposed by the U.S. against Japan to punish it for invading China. Japan's attack on Pearl Harbor was still five months in the offing, but the tension between our two countries was already high. As we sailed past the "Fuckyou Marus" the Japanese deckhands shook their fists.

Five months later, on Sunday, December 7, listening to the shocking news of Japan's attack and President Roosevelt's "day of infamy" speech on the radio, the memory of the "Fuckyou Marus" flashed through my mind. It suddenly occurred to me, sitting there stunned in my dormitory room, that if the ban on Japanese cargo ships hadn't been put into effect, one of their crews might have blown up the Panama Canal while their kamikaze brothers were decimating the U.S. fleet in Pearl Harbor.

For reasons that still perplex me, business administration, a subject that bored me silly, had been my college major. Perhaps its appeal was the special Master's degree program offered by Dartmouth's Amos Tuck School of Business that required only one postgraduate year. Or perhaps it was my memory of the armies of unemployed—talented men reduced to selling apples on street corners, their destitute families living in packing crates assembled into little cities called Hoovervilles—that made it seem important to get some practical business training. Nevertheless, I cringed at the thought of spending the rest of my years stuck behind a desk in an office.

Pearl Harbor, you could say, saved me. Because of the war, Tuck awarded us our Master's degrees three months early, in March 1942. Like most of my classmates, I immediately volunteered for the Navy's V-12 officer training program, but flunked the eye exam and was rejected. However, my less-than-20/20 vision didn't discourage the army from drafting me as a private.

Those summers spent on merchant ships did eventually lead to an unusual seafaring experience in the army. In the spring of 1943, a few months after completing Signal Corps basic training at Fort Monmouth, New Jersey, followed by Engineer Officer Candidate School at Fort Belvoir, Virginia, I was assigned to the Hampton Roads Port of Embarkation. From there the army sent me to North Africa as a cargo security officer aboard the liberty ship *John Harvard,* one of the brand-new seagoing boxes slapped together in World War II. By coincidence, the ship's captain was the former third mate of the *Floridian.*

In addition to its merchant crew, the *John Harvard* carried a navy armed guard unit to man the antiaircraft guns, as well my thirty-five-man army detachment. Our mission was to check on the tanks and armored cars stowed aboard the ship. On the return voyage we would be responsible for guarding the four hundred Italian POWs packed into the empty cargo holds, as if there was any way they could escape at sea.

Our seventy-eight ship convoy, escorted by eight or nine sub-chasers and a small aircraft carrier, crossed the Atlantic without serious incident, even though we were warned that the ocean swarmed with German submarines. On several occasions the convoy's commodore hoisted the William Fox flag, signaling the proximity of a U-boat. All the cargo ships would then maneuver evasively while the sub-chasers raced around the convoy's perimeter dropping "ashcans," as the exploding depth charges were called. "Stunning geysers erupting out of a sea that's flat as an ice rink," was the description noted in the diary that I kept every night in defiance of army regulations. It was a ridiculous rule. But the army maintained that personal diaries could provide the enemy with useful information in the event we were captured at sea.

The enlisted men in my detachment passed the long nights shooting dice and playing poker, cussing all the while that the red battle lights inside the blacked-out ship made all the cards with hearts and diamonds look like blanks. The champion crapshooter was a skinny MP from the hills of Tennessee, known simply as "Choo Choo." Each night, Choo Choo paid the messman $1.50 to serve him a full-course dinner with all the trimmings out on deck, and then promptly won back the money with a couple of rolls of the dice.

On our sixteenth night at sea, we slid past the hulking black Rock of Gibraltar and entered the Mediterranean. What had been an almost blissful Atlantic cruise suddenly became a hectic series of war exercises. Barrage balloons blossomed over the convoy, and our captain ordered everyone aboard to wear life jackets and sleep in their clothes.

We awoke the next morning to see British and American bombers circling over the convoy. A couple of fighters swooped beneath the barrage balloons, barely missing the steel cables. Once, when our ship lurched violently, we were sure we'd been hit, but it was the liberty ship off our starboard beam that had taken the torpedo. She sent up a red distress flare, then, listing to port, slowly disappeared as the convoy plodded on. We never did find out if she sank.

After three days of zigzagging across the "Med," we peeled off from the convoy and entered a pale blue harbor surrounded by a gleaming white city. "Algiers," we were finally informed. Allied ships of all shapes and sizes lay at anchor, and it quickly became clear we were engaged in the old army game of "hurry up and wait." For the next three weeks, while the casbah of Algiers beckoned temptingly in the distance, we twirled on our anchor chain, unable to go ashore. The forty-five Sherman tanks, howitzers, and crates of ammo stowed in our cargo holds might just as well have remained stored in warehouses back in Hampton Roads.

The only Algerians we encountered were the Arab bumboat boys who paddled out to trade bottles of Dago Red for cartons of Camels and Chesterfields. This was my first experience in a foreign port, and the deck-hands, all seasoned bargainers, taught me a few lessons in the art of haggling that would prove useful in Shanghai.

Wine, naturally, wasn't permitted aboard, so the bottles of Chianti were hoisted over the rail wrapped in souvenir scarves and shirts. A few bottles were reeled in on fishing lines rigged by a couple of the merchant sailors who had spotted schools of bonito chasing sardines around the harbor.

Our nights at anchor were not so idyllic. Often, we were awakened by the wail of the air-raid sirens, followed by the distant drone of the British interceptor planes taking off. A smoke screen would slowly settle over the harbor. Sometimes through the smoke we could see the orange bursts of antiaircraft shells exploding high over the city. Then, the 40mm Bofors and "Chicago pianos" would join in, scorching the blackness with thousands of red tracers. The distant thump of the pompoms added to the racket.

Usually, the protective screen of antiaircraft fire would chase the Italian bombers away, though occasionally we glimpsed the white flashes of their bombs bursting on the docks where we were waiting to unload our tanks. Searchlight beams would quickly sweep the sky seeking out the culprits. We strained to see the tiny speck of a plane where the beams converged before antiaircraft shells peppered the sky all around it—at first a little below or above, then right where the rays of light intersected. But we never did see any shells find their mark.

One night, our skywatch was diverted by an orange flare drifting silently down into the water five hundred feet off our port bow. All at once the air around our ship exploded with bursting shells. Shrapnel zinged into our wire rigging and rained down on the superstructure and hatch covers as half a dozen Italian planes roared in over the anchored cargo ships. A plume of smoke billowed from the tail of one of the Italian attackers, looking, for all the world, like a wounded plane in a Hollywood war movie.

The *John Harvard* lurched violently, then rolled gently as a bomb exploded in the water just off our stern. More bombs exploded, causing more lurches, followed by the same gentle rocking and gurgling until the ship stabilized. Our own antiaircraft guns barked into action. Several other ships joined in the free-for-all, firing a barrage of 20mm tracers that looked and sounded pretty puny compared to the heavy thudding and bright flashes of the shore batteries.

Just as unexpectedly as they came, the Italian bombers flew back out to sea. One swooped low over the *John Harvard,* giving us a farewell buzz that made everybody freeze. But the plane soared harmlessly away.

A pall of acrid smoke still hung over the harbor like an early morning mist when Sparks, our radio operator and the ship's only source of news, announced that Allied troops had landed at Messina and started up the boot of Italy. We guessed the air raid had been a retaliatory gesture, though Algiers no longer figured strategically in the war.

That didn't seem to faze the Italians. Their bombers returned several more nights before the *John Harvard* received orders to pull the hook. We then headed east along the North African coast for Bizerte, the Tunisian port known to Americans back home by the war-time hit song, "Dirty Gertie from Bizerte." And there we finally did get ashore for one day.

At that time, Bizerte displayed an odd mixture of traditional Muslim, ancient Roman, French colonial, and American military trappings. It was my first exposure to the clash of ancient and modern cultures that a few years later would hit me so hard in Shanghai. In Bizerte it was camel caravans plodding alongside convoys of armored cars, or Arab peddlers spreading out their wares in the shade of an old Roman viaduct, or little pockmarked girl pimps offering sex with their mothers for $2 U.S.

On a whirlwind sightseeing tour of nearby Carthage, I tried to cover as many of the historic landmarks and absorb as much of the local culture as was possible. The two main attractions were the Antonine Baths, once the largest in the Roman Empire, and the ancient Tophet graveyard, with its rows of tiny headstones where child sacrifices were performed. However, as my Arab guide explained, the softhearted Carthaginians usually substituted

lambs or kid goats, or even dead children, for the live boys and girls scheduled to be beheaded.

The *John Harvard*'s captain was wise to have granted that brief, one-day
shore leave. By then everybody aboard ship had come down with a bad case
of cabin fever, adding to the inherent friction between the navy armed guards
and the merchant sailors, who kept bragging about the $150 bonus they
were being paid for every air raid. The bad feeling had finally boiled over into
a fistfight during one of the daily poker games on the forward hatch. It took
an infusion of joy spread by the "Wop POWs," as we called the four hundred Italian prisoners jammed into the cargo holds, to break the tension.
Deliriously happy to be out of the war, they broke out their accordions and
guitars and serenaded the ship with Italian love songs all the way back to the
Hampton Roads Port of Embarkation. There, the prisoners were deloused
and sent off, still singing, to detention camps in the Midwest, where they remained until the end of the war.

After that forty-five-day round-trip and tiny taste of Africa, I volunteered for a permanent overseas assignment. Many of my fellow officers who
enjoyed cushy jobs at Hampton Roads thought it was a crazy idea. But by
then I had been promoted to first lieutenant, and army life in the U.S.
seemed unbearably bureaucratic. Besides, most of my classmates at officers'
candidate school had already shipped out to the Pacific.

The Pacific war was expanding rapidly. Even so, it took three months
for my request to be acted on. Finally, in November 1943, I found myself
headed for New Guinea aboard the army transport *General J. H. McRae*,
packed with three thousand members of the Mississippi National Guard.
My twenty cabin mates all had nicknames like "Possum," "Gray Squirrel,"
and "Woodchuck." There didn't seem to be a Tom, Dick, or Harry among
them. Their patois was no more understandable than the pidgin English
of the native Papuans, or "Fuzzy Wuzzies," who with their frizzy yellow hair
(dyed with dissolved Atabrine tablets) and brown betel nut-stained teeth,
greeted us with big smiles at the replacement depot, or "repple-depple" as it
was known, in Oro Bay.

Once again, it was hurry up and wait. The war was still far away, and our main diversion came from watching the Fuzzy Wuzzies catch fish (*hukim pis* in pidgin). Standing on the shore in the late afternoon (*apinun*), they would hurl hand grenades out into the rolling surf. The underwater blast would sometimes kill an entire school, leaving the dead fish to wash belly-up onto the beach, which the Fuzzy Wuzzies would then barbecue (*kukim long*) over an open fire. But the most eagerly awaited event in the repple-depple was our weekly ration of beer—limited to one tropically-heated can, which some enterprising soul discovered could be pleasantly chilled by spraying it with mosquito repellent. The freon gas in the aerosol bomb served as a cooling agent.

It was late December by the time the army sent us by supply ship up the coast of New Guinea to Hollandia, on the next leg of a drawn-out journey to the war. We enjoyed Christmas dinner there at a tent camp nicknamed "Hotel Piztoff" before being flown on to Peleliu Island and another tent camp called the Peleliu Palace. Although the Marines had pretty well cleaned out the atoll's coral caves in bloody hand-to-hand combat, a few Japanese remained in hiding. From Peleliu it was on to Leyte Island in the Philippines and another replacement depot, this one consisting solely of foxholes dug amongst the coconut palms because of the Japs' nightly air raids. The war was finally getting closer.

At last, on February 1, 1944, my twenty-fourth birthday, we landed at Lingayen Gulf in northern Luzon. Still classified as replacements, though temporarily attached to the Fourth Engineer Special Brigade, we slogged south for Manila. The Filipino men, women, and children in the barrios along the highway cheered, offering us bunches of bananas and coconut milk as we passed by. I was captivated by these handsome, soft-spoken Orientals, nicknamed our "little brown brothers," after the U.S. acquired the Philippines as Spanish–American War booty. Looking back, I guess it was on the road to Manila that I first fell in love with Asia, a deep affection that would haunt me forever.

The Japanese still occupied the post office and several other buildings in Manila when we arrived. The city crackled with sporadic sniper fire, although the heavy fighting was over. Hundreds of wrecked Japanese cargo ships—Fuckyou Marus, I still called them—with only a bow or stern sticking up out of the water, dotted the harbor. A few crew members remained aboard the derelicts, refusing to surrender. When their food and water finally ran out, they committed hara-kiri, or hung themselves, their sun-shriveled corpses left swinging from the rigging.

Much to my disappointment, I was first put to work in General MacArthur's headquarters. My journalism experience at Dartmouth had somehow crept into my army personnel file, resulting in an assignment to write press releases describing the heroics of the conquering G.I.s for their hometown newspapers. But as preparations for the invasion of Japan started to take shape, I was pulled off that boring press release detail and put in command of a DUKW (landing craft) company based in the Passig River, which separates modern Manila from Intramuros, the old Spanish section.

That duty lasted for a year. The hardest part of the assignment was maintaining discipline among the enlisted men, who quickly discovered the cadre of Filipina hookers hanging around the port. Our PX supplies, especially cigarettes, also had a way of disappearing into the city's black market aboard the boxy, wheeled *DUKWs* that could run on land, as well as in water.

In August 1945, we were busy loading supply ships for the invasion of Japan when the two atomic bombs incinerated Hiroshima and Nagasaki, precipitating Japan's sudden surrender. The U.S Army in the Philippines was also caught by surprise. From then until the following February thousands of us were stranded in Manila. Frustrated by the lack of troop transports to carry us back across the Pacific, we stamped NO BOATS, NO VOTES on the envelopes of our letters sent home, hoping that might goad Congress into taking some action to speed up our return. As the months slipped by, I briefly considered taking my discharge in Manila and heading directly for China. But my father had died a year earlier, and it seemed important to return to New York City first to visit my mother.

The boring days and nights in Manila with few duties to perform provided ample time to plot a postwar career. My ambition to become a foreign correspondent hadn't dimmed. If anything, it had turned into an obsession. It wasn't simply the glamor of the job or the desire to travel, but a gnawing curiosity about the world's political leaders whose charisma or cunning enabled them to alter history. I had spent hours dissecting the profiles of Stalin, Hitler, and Roosevelt that appeared in the shrunk-down pony editions of *Time* magazine, trying to figure out what it was that made each of those men so powerful.

In due course sufficient troop ships were mobilized to repatriate everybody. Marching up the gangplank of the *Marine Swallow*, I felt a sudden wave of nostalgia for Asia. It was nice to be going home. But at the same time, I hated to leave that part of the world. Those mixed feelings were only partially relieved by what turned out to be a sodden voyage to San Francisco.

Liquor, of course, was prohibited on all army transports. But it came aboard the *Marine Swallow* by the case, hidden in backpacks, laundry bags, and duffels. My twenty-sixth birthday occurred halfway across the Pacific and the party to mark that occasion went on for two days. We were all ready to call it quits after the first night's festivities. But as the sun's first rays peeked through the porthole, one of my cabinmates pointed out that we had just crossed the international date line and another February 1 was dawning, which also had to be celebrated.

Arriving back in the U.S., I traveled cross-country by train to the Fort Dix hospital in New Jersey to be checked and rechecked for any lingering traces of malaria. The Atabrine pills that turned all of our skins yellow in New Guinea and the Philippines merely suppressed the symptoms we suffered periodically. In any case, I now felt fine. So at night my hospital roommate and I would slip out of bed and hop a train for New York City, where we tried, or so it seemed, to see who could consume the most beer. The malaria symptoms finally disappeared—cured, my roommate claimed, by the nightly doses of hops and malt—and the army discharged me.

The next two months turned into a nonstop assault on the newspapers, magazines, and all three wire services in New York City. "Send me anywhere," I told a vast array of editors, "though I'd prefer an assignment in China."

That last request elicited a wry smile and a gentle reminder that quite a few veteran war correspondents, cooling their heels on dull domestic assignments, were also eager to go back to the Far East. Barry Farris, the curmudgeonly gruff general manager of the International News Service, did take pity on me and proposed a rewrite assignment in Atlanta, but warned that the job was probably a dead end. In spite of all the turndowns, a reporting job in China still loomed large in my sights.

One of my former army commanders had suggested that if all else failed, I might want to apply for a copywriting job in the advertising department at Remington Rand, where he had worked before the war. As a last resort I did apply. And much to my surprise, or to be truthful, horror, was immediately hired. The thought of spending years grinding out prose about the virtues of Remington typewriters was not appealing. But I needed a job.

A few days before starting work, a friend spotted a newspaper article announcing that UNRRA was recruiting men and women for work in China and Ethiopia. That night, an army buddy from the Philippines and I were trying to drown my sorrows about the Remington Rand job, when we both suddenly decided to send telegrams offering our services to UNRRA. The next morning, still a little fuzzy from the previous night's consumption of beer, bourbon, and wine, we awoke with the vague feeling that we had done something important. But neither of us could immediately recall what it was. By late afternoon a return telegram came from UNRRA inviting us to come down to Washington, D.C. for interviews.

UNRRA, apparently, was desperate. Because of my wartime experience with DUKWs ("They're like trucks aren't they?" said the personnel man), I was immediately offered a job in China as a transportation specialist. Without giving it a second thought, I accepted. My buddy, an artillery battery commander, was not so lucky. But as a consolation prize he was offered an administrative post in Ethiopia, which he turned down. So without having done a day's work for Remington Rand, I telephoned the company and resigned.

There were about fifty UNRRA recruits destined for China. We were given a one-month orientation course, including some basic lessons in spoken Chinese. On July 5, after crossing the country by train, we boarded a chartered Pacific Overseas Airways DC-4 in Ontario, California, bound for Shanghai. The flight across the Pacific was a ten-thousand-mile, 120-hour odyssey, with everyone strapped into metal bucket seats. I remember the plane seemed to be droning on forever above the placid blue ocean, interspersed by refueling stops at Honolulu, Johnston Atoll, Kwajelein, and Guam. About the only break in the monotony came during our departure from Johnston Atoll, a tropical speck of land almost entirely populated by "gooney birds," as the black-footed albatrosses were called.

Over the intercom, our pilot informed us that a flock of gooney birds flying into the propellers of a four-engine transport like ours could bring the plane down as effectively as a barrage of antiaircraft artillery. That's why, he explained, an army jeep was speeding down the runway ahead of our plane during takeoff, shooing the gooney birds away. Finally, on July 11, 1946, after a day lost crossing the international dateline, we taxied up to the dilapidated terminal at Shanghai's Kiangwan Airport.

2

THE KINGDOM OF SQUEEZE

UNRRA, it quickly became apparent, knew the hurry-up-and-wait game as well as the U.S. Army. For a week all the new recruits drifted around Shanghai with no work to do. Our superiors hadn't yet figured out where to assign us. Or perhaps in my case they wondered why the former commander of an army DUKW company had been hired in the first place. Whatever the reason, nobody seemed to care that we were enjoying a paid vacation.

For brand-new China-hands the city was nonstop theater. We explored the various side alleys, loitered in the teahouses, sniffed the pungent food stalls, and pored over the myriad souvenir shops piled high with carved ivory knickknacks, from Buddhas to backscratchers. Once, defying the imperious stare of the gold-epauletted Chinese doorman, a couple of us risked poking our heads inside the exclusive, all-male Shanghai Club, boasting the longest bar in the world. And for luck, we followed the locals' example and rubbed the shiny paws of the two larger-than-life bronze lions guarding the Hong Kong and Shanghai Bank. Those two symbols of power and prosperity, both males, we were told, "roar when a virgin rubs their paws." But because there are no virgins in Shanghai, they remained silent.

Our orientation lectures in Washington had touched on the origins of the Chinese Communist Party. So some of us made it a point to locate the old schoolhouse on Rue Beyle in the French Concession where Mao Zedong and the other organizers held their first meeting in 1921. Then, for the women in our group, there was Yates Road, known to British matrons as "the street of a thousand nighties," where they could buy everything at great discounts.

The Great World amusement center fascinated me as the most un-Chinese monstrosity in this part-Western, part-Oriental city. Encircled by balconies and topped with a tall minaret, the seedy six-story fun house catered mainly to coolies with but a few pennies to spend on entertainment. Yet, I found it hard to pass by without peeking in at the circus-mix of magicians, puppets, clowns, jugglers, fortune-tellers, acrobats, patent medicine vendors—even earwax extractors. In its heyday before World War II, the Great World was a notorious vice mecca. A British gentleman was said to have harrumphed, "No male can walk through the place without feeling female hands tugging at his elbow." But the most famous bordello frequented over the years by Brits was the Vice Consulate, where it was said that "diplomatic relations were carried out horizontally."

Those early explorations of the city were shared with Mildred Gokey, an attractive twenty-five-year-old UNRRA woman who had flown over to Shanghai on the same plane. She had worked as a secretary for the relief agency in Washington before wangling the overseas assignment. We seemed to have the same thirst for adventure, the same curiosity about China, and the same hunger for companionship. Soon it was more than that. After spending four years in the army's almost all-male environment, I found Millie's bright smile and quick mind irresistible.

After the week we spent touring Shanghai together, I was finally given a job. Much to my surprise it was not with UNRRA, but with the China National Relief and Rehabilitation Administration, CNRRA, the international relief agency's Chinese counterpart. "Welcome, mate," an Australian sanitary engineer already working there greeted me. "Welcome to the kingdom of squeeze."

"Squeeze? What's that?" I asked. The word had never come up in our orientation lectures.

"Cumshaw, kickbacks, graft, whatever you want to call the petty-fucking-larceny extracted by functionaries up and down the fucking CNRRA supply chain!" he exclaimed with the usual Aussie abundance of expletives. He then related how T. V. Soong, Chiang Kai-shek's powerful financier brother-in-law, had stipulated in writing that "to preserve the dignity of the Chinese people," all UNRRA supplies had to be placed under China's control as soon as they reached Shanghai.

"It's a matter of face," added the Aussie. "Something you'll soon understand." Still, it didn't make much sense since all of the relief programs in the country were being run by Americans or the by other foreign nationals employed by UNRRA. But apparently Soong had persisted, and that's how CNRRA came into being.

At the time, I was too ignorant of the corruption plaguing Chiang Kai-shek's Nationalist regime to appreciate Soong's real reason for adding another bureaucratic layer to the relief operation. The Aussie admitted that nobody dared estimate how much of the $685 million worth of food, clothing, and equipment turned over to CNRRA was going directly into the black market.

My initial assignment was to develop a plan for reducing the pilferage of UNRRA shipments arriving at Shanghai's crowded port. I was given my own tugboat with a Chinese crew of three to cruise up and down the Huangpu River. Part of the job was to make sure the poor, perspiring coolies, chanting "ai-ho, ai-ho" as they struggled under their heavy loads, weren't swiping handfuls of rice, flour, or anything else. What a farce. No coolie would have dared steal a grain of rice for fear of being brutally beaten by his stevedore boss and tossed semiconscious into the river. The real thievery, of course, was being conducted at a much higher, unseen level. It was an open secret that CNRRA's top brass was squeezing a 10-percent kickback out of every ton of UNRRA cargo handled by the privately owned stevedoring companies.

The chaos of Shanghai's waterfront was hard to believe—far worse than was Manila's congested harbor when we were preparing to invade Japan. At night, nested along the docks and godowns (warehouses) lining the Huangpu and jammed into the adjoining Suzhou Creek, were more than one hundred thousand sampans, junks, lighters, barges, and ancient arks of all shapes and sizes—a floating city within the city. These small boats served as bedroom, kitchen, nursery, and old-age home for a vast population that used the polluted waters for bathing, laundry, and toilet.

At dawn, the entire armada would move out into the harbor to ferry passengers, unload the hulking foreign freighters, load the rusting coastal steamers, or simply barter Chinese souvenirs for American cigarettes with the sailors aboard the U.S. and British warships. A few sampans prowled the river scavenging for garbage dumped overboard by the foreign passenger liners.

The smallest of these native vessels were propelled by a giant oar wiggled back and forth from the stern; the larger craft by a putt-putting, exhaust-belching diesel. While the man-of-the-boat steered or wrestled cargo, his wife mended clothes or cooked the family's meals in a huge cauldron on the stern. Their "creek children," as they were called, were either tethered to the mast or tended by grandma, while grandpa smoked his long pipe up in the bow. Births, deaths, marriages, and all superstitious rites were performed afloat. So, except to take on fuel or fresh water, there was little reason for the citizens of this vast water-borne community to go ashore.

One of my first purchases in Shanghai was a secondhand Japanese Minoltaflex camera. This cheap copy of a German Rolleiflex cost thirty-five dollars "U.S.," as we used to say to avoid confusion with prices quoted in Chinese yuan. For a buck at the same photo supply store, I picked up a frayed book on how to take news pictures written by Kip Ross, photo editor of the *National Geographic*. While making my rounds on the CNRRA tug, both of these purchases were put to good use shooting a photo essay on the squalid life of the boat people. But what to do with this story? After much hesitation, I sent the prints, captions, and accompanying article, titled "Sampan City," off to Kip Ross at the *Geographic,* expecting nothing more than a note of encouragement from some lowly clerk in the photo department.

Several months later, a check for forty-five dollars arrived from the magazine. A note signed simply "Kip" explained that while he couldn't use the story, he was purchasing the rights to nine of my photographs as "stock" for possible future use in some other story. Deducting the cost of the camera and book, I had already made a profit of nine dollars.

Another dividend from my harbor surveillance job was a flurry of invitations to Sunday brunches traditionally held on the wharves of the various foreign shipping companies. These magnificent buffets, it seemed, had come down to a contest to see which company could serve the hottest Indian curry, one that would leave your tongue scorched and your throat on fire. Gulping water didn't help. But choking down a banana did bring temporary relief. According to my scalded mouth, the clear winner was the Jardine, Matheson and Company, which claimed to have been perfecting its curry recipe for a hundred years, ever since the firm's two Scottish founders, William Jardine and James Matheson, started smuggling opium into Shanghai.

On one of my surveillance runs I was excited to see the *Floridian,* the American Hawaii Line rust-pot I had worked on, steam into Shanghai all dolled up in a fresh coat of paint. Its cargo holds were filled with bales of used clothing earmarked for UNRRA. Nudging my tug alongside, I climbed up the Jacob's ladder hoping to find a least one familiar face. No luck. The ship now carried a Filipino crew. But I did locate the tiny two-bunk, single-porthole cabin I shared with Ned, the other wiper. Ned and I had planned to jump ship in San Francisco, buy an old rattletrap, and drive back across the country. But while the ship was getting its bottom painted in dry dock in Oakland, someone slipped into our cabin and stole the four crisp twenty-dollar bills each of us had just been paid. That was my first encounter with a thief, and I could still feel the fury of losing all the sweat-money earned working down in the *Floridian*'s sweltering 120-degree engine room. Flat broke and forced to remain on board for the three-week return voyage through the Panama Canal, I remember standing on the fantail and forlornly watching the Golden Gate Bridge disappear over the horizon. I felt cheated, robbed of a scenic trip across the country.

Six years later, standing on the fantail again, I watched the bales of used clothing being hoisted out of the hold and dropped into sampans that ferried them ashore. Well, if all this used clothing ends up in the black market and never reaches the peasants for whom it was intended, at least they won't feel cheated as I had. They'll never know it was meant for them.

As my Australian colleague at CNRRA predicted, my job proved to be more frustrating than fun. On another surveillance trip aboard the tug I spotted a number of pallets loaded with crates of automotive parts being whisked away by trucks that didn't belong to CNRRA. I reported this irregularity to Mr. Li, my immediate superior. "Don't worry about it," he said. "Not all of our trucks have the CNRRA insignia stenciled on them."

After voicing my suspicions to one of the higher-ups in UNRRA, Mr. Li summoned me to CNRRA headquarters. A cadre of Chinese clerks, all clad in blue gowns, were, as usual, sipping their tea and furiously clicking their abacuses in the outer office. Finally, led into Mr. Li's inner sanctum, I was informed that he thought my skills could be better used escorting CNRRA freight trains to the interior. Too many CNRRA trains, he claimed, were being commandeered by either the Communist or Nationalist armies. As always, Mr. Li was unctuously polite, praising me for doing such a fine job patrolling the riverfront. No mention was made of my tattletailing to UNRRA, though undoubtedly that was what had precipitated the change in my assignment.

"The railway job will be much more challenging," he assured me. "Part of the time you will be operating in a war zone." Then he added, "But as a former army officer I'm sure you won't mind that."

I didn't mind the change. Up until then my spare-time travels with Millie had been confined to Shanghai's suburbs. The new job, although still under Mr. Li's supervision, would provide an opportunity to observe the interior countryside from slow-moving boxcars. And as he also pointed out, "You will get to visit a number of ancient cities."

Silly as it sounds, aside from being away from Millie for weeks at a time, my only reluctance was the loss of my position as starting pitcher on UNRRA's baseball team. After being so suddenly immersed in an alien culture, playing baseball was a reassuring link to life in America. Besides, we were battling for first place in the Shanghai City League, comprised of former military personnel. I also suspected that the train job, aside from getting me out of Mr. Li's hair, might be another form of make-work concocted by CNRRA to keep us Americans busy. Anyway, it would have been pointless to refuse to go.

A few days later, I was clanking along the bumpy roadbed en route to Bengpu, an important market town and rail center in Anhui Province. My instructions from Mr. Li were brief, but specific: "Make sure the entire train reaches Bengpu intact. And then returns to Shanghai intact." But what in the world was I supposed to do if the soldiers of one army or the other ransacked the cargo or, worse yet, took off with the entire train? Not much help could be expected from the three sleepy-eyed armed guards—"Hear-No-Evil," "See-No-Evil," and "Speak-No-Evil"—lounging back in the caboose.

Also accompanying me were four young Chinese cargo supervisors. We slept in the same boxcar, using sacks of flour—our main cargo—for pillows. They boarded the train empty-handed, but bought eggs, rice, and sweet potatoes from the shouting and gesturing vendors lining the station platforms. My contribution to our combined larder was a full case of U.S. Army Ten-in-One Rations, which handily also contained toilet paper, water purification tablets, and cigarettes. One of the cargo supervisors, cooking everything mixed together over glowing coals in an empty bucket, produced some very tasty Chinese fare.

The seven-hundred-mile round-trip was scheduled to take ten days—three days each way and four days to unload. This timetable, it quickly became evident, was totally unrealistic because of numerous unscheduled stops and the snail's pace of the train when it was underway. But that didn't matter. I had brought the camera along, and the verdant, manicured farmland, heavily veined with rivers and canals, proved to be a photographer's paradise. Many times the canals weren't visible, only the colorful batwing sails of the junks sticking up out of the fields. Irrigating the farm plots were small picturesque pumping stations, powered usually by donkeys or oxen, or sometimes by women. The train itself was also very photogenic. Hundreds of peasants, together with their children, pigs, and chickens, clung to the roof of the boxcars and cowcatcher of the locomotive, emerging from the tunnels with their faces covered with soot.

Arriving at the halfway point in Nanjing (Nanking), the freight cars were uncoupled and loaded one by one onto a ferry that carried them across the Yangtze River to Pukow, where the train was then reassembled. "How could this antique ferry stay afloat under the weight of a train?" I wondered. Only recently, the English-language *Shanghai Evening Post and Mercury* had run a story about an overloaded passenger ferry that had capsized making this same river crossing, drowning more than four hundred men, women, and children. Apparently, all of the people aboard rushed to one side as the boat approached the dock, causing it to flip over. But then, according to the newspaper, capsizing ferries were an all-too-common occurrence in China.

We pulled into Bengpu in the black of night. Mr. Li had advised my staying at the Jesuit mission run by a group of Italian fathers. He scrawled the directions to the mission in Chinese. But none of the rickshaw boys parked at the station could read. An old gentleman came to my rescue and told one of them where to go. Suddenly, I was lurching through a maze of narrow lantern-lit streets, past shuttered shops, soon to be delivered, I suspected, to the lair of some knife-wielding bandit, who would relieve me of all my money. You've seen too many Fu Man Chu movies, I reminded myself. This is the real China. Not the Hollywood version.

The bearded missionaries turned out to be most hospitable, and also highly knowledgeable about Bengpu and the surrounding Anhui countryside. By the time I arrived they had finished supper and were chanting evening prayers in the big redbrick church. "You are welcome to share our food and shelter," offered Bishop Cassini, who then instructed Brother John to escort me to a spartan, cell-sized room containing a washbowl, a chamber pot, and the portrait of some unrecognizable saint staring benevolently down from the wall. But the most welcome sight of all was a cot with clean sheets.

Early the next morning, Father Minella, as he introduced himself in fluent English, suggested that we bicycle together on his rounds to the neighboring villages and farms. He promised to show me the beautiful pomegranate orchards that once belonged to the Ming Dynasty emperors. Everywhere we went, riding along the top of the Huai River dikes from one small cluster of mud huts to another, it was I, not Father Minella, who was the main attraction. The peasants there had never met an American before. In fact, most of them had no idea where or what America was. They asked such simple questions as, "Does it rain there?" and "Do you have boats as big as our junks?"

Reaching a tributary of the Huai, we squeezed our bikes into a sampan already filled with patiently waiting passengers. One of the farmers had brought along two cows, which he had tied to a rope so they could swim alongside the sampan. The river crossing proceeded smoothly enough until we hit a sand bar and the cows began walking around in circles in the shallow water, turning the sampan with them like the hands of a clock. Finally, much to the glee of his fellow passengers, the cows' owner peeled off his clothes and jumped into the water with the two beasts to keep them pointed in the right direction.

Father Minella, a handsome, energetic fifty-year-old, proved to be an engrossing companion. He had trained in Rome for the prescribed fourteen years to become a Jesuit priest, before joining the mission in Bengpu. A very humble man in his dealings with the local citizenry, he was different from the missionaries I'd encountered in Shanghai. They, like so many foreign businessmen, didn't seem to think of themselves as guests to be tolerated, but as benefactors without whom the Chinese could barely exist.

In Bengpu, Father Minella realized he had to first win the people's trust and friendship before beginning the almost hopeless task of converting them to Christianity. Later, as we traveled down the main river, stretched out in the sun on the deck of a steamboat, he confided his frustration of trying to interest confirmed Buddhists in Catholicism. I became aware of the boat's undersized engine struggling against the swift current just as this priest was struggling to explain his mixed emotions about trying to carry out God's work.

"Many who do convert, I fear, are 'rice Christians,'" he admitted, indicating that he suspected the mission's handouts of free food had probably won them over. "It's not that I consider these peasants heathens," he added, "not in a land dotted with pagodas, temples and other Chinese places of worship."

"Why don't you give up the priesthood, or at least request a transfer to another country?" I asked, but immediately felt silly offering such flip suggestions to a man sworn to celibacy and willingly undergoing so many other deprivations in China.

Father Minella was appalled. "Give up!" he exclaimed. "Our church has been in Bengpu for centuries. We are not here only to spread the word of God and save souls. Our responsibility is much broader. We teach sanitation, and modern agriculture, and many other practical things. I expect to stay here until I die."

"And if the Communists capture Bengpu. What then?" I asked.

"The people in Bengpu are farmers and shopkeepers, not Communists or Nationalists," he replied. "I will remain here, just as I did during the Japanese occupation."

When it came time for me to escort the empty train back to Shanghai, the boxcars were already jammed with wounded Nationalist soldiers. Mr. Li had warned me that this might happen. Evidently, it was CNRRA's policy to provide free transportation home for these pitifully mutilated men, most of them baring crudely amputated arms or legs, or bandaged heads still oozing blood. I was informed that this particular group came from the neighboring province of Henan, victims of a hit-and-run attack by the "One-Eyed Dragon," as the much-feared Communist general Liu Bocheng was known.

Ten days later, the rail journey to Bengpu had to be repeated, once more with the same cargo of flour. But this time I also brought along boxes of American magazines to give to Father Minella and the other priests at the mission. Isabella Van Meter Leland, formerly Henry Luce's assistant in New York and the wife of UNRRA's deputy medical director in China who, coincidentally, was Millie's boss, served as the business manager of the Time–Life bureau in Shanghai. She was delighted to get rid of all the back issues cluttering her office. And I was delighted to deliver them to the Fathers who so kindly provided me with hot meals and a clean bed.

Two memorable occurrences marked the second trip to Bengpu. Our steam locomotive disappeared, leaving the empty boxcars stranded on a siding for three days. It was never determined whose army—Mao's or Chiang's—stole it. Then, while awaiting a replacement engine, Anhui's jovial provincial governor tossed an enormous banquet to celebrate the anniversary of V-J Day—complete with brass band, mountains of Chinese delicacies served on white tablecloths, and silver goblets of hot rice wine to wash everything down. But as I wrote to my friends back home, "All of the mandarins, mayors and other high muckymucks present, belched, regurgitated, blew their collective noses, spat on the floor, and made other unsavory noises throughout the meal." I also voiced suspicions in those letters that the money for this magnificent feast probably came from my host selling some of the CNRRA flour that was being delivered by train to Bengpu.

As the only *gweilo* (foreigner) present at the banquet, I was singled out by the governor as the guest of honor. My grungy suntans and unkempt appearance after several nights in the boxcar didn't seem to matter. As the honored guest, the only thing that mattered was that I toast everyone present with *bai-gar,* the fiery white liquor distilled from *gaoliang* (sorghum). It was one *gambei* (bottoms up) after another until I left the banquet with a skull-rattling headache and legs so wobbly the rickshaw boy had a hard time keeping me from falling out of his conveyance during the ride back to the mission. Practicing a little temperance at future banquets, I learned to surreptitiously spill half the contents of each freshly poured porcelain cup of white lightning under the table.

My railway escort duties kept taking me deeper and deeper into the interior, where misty mountains rose out of the Central Plain. It may have been happenstance, or it could have been that Mr. Li and his boss, Mr. K. Y. Chen, wanted to keep me out of the CNRRA office in Shanghai for longer and longer periods of time. The black marketing of CNRRA supplies was becoming ever more flagrant, and the two men eyed me and the other Americans working for them as potential whistle-blowers. It took a while for me to realize that the whole concept of charity—especially a giveaway program administered by an international relief organization—was completely alien to the Chinese. Handing out free food, clothing, and agricultural equipment was simply incomprehensible. Besides, according to Chinese tradition, continuing responsibilities were connected to any charitable act. Even if you happened upon an injured person gushing blood in the street, you'd better think twice before offering assistance for fear of having to care for that person forever.

Only occasionally did UNRRA take any action against the wholesale plundering of its relief supplies. Once, when it was discovered that blood plasma donated by the American Red Cross was being sold in Shanghai drugstores for twenty-five dollars a pint, UNRRA ordered the U.S. Navy shore patrol to seize the 3,500 cases still stored in the godown.

Another time it was a shipload of war-surplus jeeps that had to be recovered. But in this case the jeeps all had traceable serial numbers, preventing CNRRA from peddling them through local car dealers. But that wasn't the end of it. Miffed at missing out on a hefty piece of black market business, the car dealers got the Nationalist government to lodge an official protest. It accused the U.S. of dumping free vehicles on the local market and requested that, henceforth, UNRRA buy all of its jeeps from Chinese dealers before turning them over to CNRRA. The stench of that proposal carried all the way back to Washington, where it was flatly rejected. Most of the time, however, UNRRA simply refused to act, claiming corruption was too deeply rooted in the Nationalist regime to do anything about.

Whatever Mr. Li's reason was for sending me off to such remote cities as Wuhan, Xian, and Zhengzhou, I was delighted with the chance to see more of China. My duties had also changed. I was now charged, in effect, with lassoing dozens of lost locomotives and hundreds of lost boxcars, like a cowboy rounding up stray cattle. To do this I had to enlist the help of the managing director of both the east–west Lunghai line and north–south Ping-Han line.

Traveling with these Chinese bigwigs in their private railway cars turned out to be a moveable feast.

At every station the railway workers and their families waited in formation to greet the director. And at the main stops his private car was purposely shunted off to a siding so he and his entourage could be feted with a twenty- or thirty-course banquet—squab, sharks' fins, duck, lobster, doves' eggs, bird's nest soup, and those seemingly inescapable tiny, live freshwater shrimp, served at every banquet in a covered dish so they couldn't jump out.

I finally learned that the prescribed way of eating those critters was to snag one with the chopsticks, dip it in the spicy sauce provided to both enhance the taste and anesthetize the shrimp, then bite its head off before swallowing. Occasionally forgetting the decapitation step, I could feel the shrimp wriggling all the way down to my stomach. But the most memorable dish of all was a Henan Province specialty called "living fish." While the guests clapped appreciatively, a Yellow River carp was dipped tail-first in boiling oil and then smothered in sweet and sour sauce, before being delivered to the table with its unscalded gills and mouth still opening and closing.

The Chinese, I knew, had a strong appetite for certain live animals—proof that the meat was fresh. Monkey brains were considered a Guangzhou (Canton) specialty. A round table with a deep cavity in the middle was used to contain the kicking and screeching simian. Then the top of the poor creature's skull was peeled back to bare its warm brains, permitting the diners to pick away with their chopsticks. Fortunately, I never had to endure that delicacy.

Most of the train trips were far from luxurious. Even first class meant sharing a sleeping car compartment with five others, usually high-ranking Nationalist army officers traveling with their wives and children. Between their snoring, slurping, smoking, chewing of watermelon seeds, and singsong chattering, carried on throughout the day and far into the night, sleep was hard to come by. Nevertheless, the close quarters forced me to practice speaking Mandarin. And the spectacular mountain and river views kept me shooting roll after roll of black-and-white film and filling my notebooks with vivid first impressions.

My original plan was to write a series of descriptive articles about this populous, war-torn land once called the Middle Kingdom symbolized by a dragon—that fire-breathing, mythical creature the Chinese considered both powerful and benevolent. But on the protracted train rides, I started toying instead with the idea of an exposé titled "UNRRA in Bandit Land." Before leaving New York, I had made arrangements to send any serious writing endeavors to the mother of a friend of mine, a freelance editor who also worked as a part-time literary agent. So I sent her a letter describing what I had in mind.

"You see," I wrote, "Chiang Kai-shek persists in referring to the Communist soldiers as 'bandits' and to his own troops as 'bandit suppression forces.' And here am I, in the midst of these military bandits and their suppressors, working for high-level CNRRA bandits, who keep sending me off to recover stolen rolling stock while they stay back in Shanghai stealing all the relief supplies they can get their hands on. Believe me, a really scathing article is taking shape in my mind."

The letter was probably overly irate, but it proceeded to explain that those angry thoughts were unavoidable on rail journeys plagued by dynamited trestles, uprooted rails, and mangled switches destroyed during Communist hit-and-run attacks or Nationalist counterattacks. "It was no surprise," I explained, "when a train shuddered to a stop and the passengers stoically disembarked, only to wait for another train to appear at the other side of the break, which could take an hour or a day. Under those conditions, a scheduled three-day express trip from Shanghai to Xian might last a week or more." To drive home the point, I ended the letter by asking, "How would Americans behave if they had to suffer those trials and tribulations on a trip of about the same distance from New York to St. Louis?"

From her return letter, it was clear she didn't have a clue about what was going on in China. Nevertheless, she urged me to tackle the exposé and to send it to her as soon as I could. The *Nation,* a liberal muckraking publication, she thought, might be interested. With that article in mind, I embarked on future rail journeys with renewed energy and increased note-taking.

Xian was the westernmost terminus of my travels. Situated in a fertile cotton-and-wheat-growing basin in Shaanxi Province, it had been the capital of all China during the Han, Xin, Zhou, and Tang dynasties. And as a result, the city was sprinkled with ancient drum towers, bell towers, palaces, and temples left by the former emperors. But it was only after the unearthing of the army of life-size terra-cotta soldiers in 1965 that Xian became a tourist mecca.

The sooty old rail yard bore no special trappings, though it was the largest and most difficult to contend with in my search for missing locomotives and boxcars. After a week of that exhausting and dirty work, I declared a one-day holiday. No excuse for a day off was really needed because it was Chiang Kai-shek's birthday, and all the railway workers, whose help I required, were off ringing gongs, exploding firecrackers, or getting drunk.

First, I stopped in at the local bathhouse and ordered the full treatment: camphor oil rubdown, manicure, pedicure, massage, bath, and shampoo, interspersed with rest periods for drinking tea and chewing watermelon seeds. Only when the in-house acupuncturist began brandishing his long needles did I decline one of the proffered services.

The rest of my day was spent sightseeing and looking for background material for the exposé. I even managed to locate the infamous Tiger Rock, where in 1936 Generalissimo Chiang Kai-shek was captured by his own drug-addicted deputy commander in chief, Zhang Xueliang, known as the "Young Marshal." In what came to be called the Xian Incident, members of the Young Marshal's Elite Corps had shot their way into the Palace of Glorious Purity, where the Generalissimo was spending the night, killing his nephew. But that was only the beginning of one of the wildest stories recorded in China's political history.

When the shooting occurred, Chiang was doing his morning exercises in front of an open window. He jumped out, climbed the palace wall, fell in a ditch, and then squeezed himself into a crevice in Tiger Rock, where he was captured a few hours later. Barefoot and still dressed in his pajamas, he was also minus his dentures and couldn't speak.

Mao received the unexpected good news with great excitement. "Chiang owes us a blood debt high as a mountain!" he exclaimed. But cooler Communist heads prevailed, especially Zhou Enlai's, thus preventing the Nationalist leader's execution. Held prisoner for two weeks, Chiang was finally released, but only after agreeing to the Young Marshal's demand that his Nationalist troops fight side by side with the Communists in a united front against the Japanese.

This epic tale, however, didn't end there. In an ironic twist, the Generalissimo was escorted safely back to Nanjing by the Young Marshal, who was immediately imprisoned after making the mistake of surrendering to atone for the betrayal of his leader. "I did what I thought was best for China," said the Young Marshal. "And now I stand before you. Do with me what you will."

Despite the Generalissimo's promise, his armies never did fight very spiritedly alongside the Communists against the Japanese. And the Young Marshal ended up with Chiang in Taiwan, where he remained under house arrest, "besotted by opium and weakened by concubines," according to one report.

Wherever the hunt for the lost rolling stock took me, I heard horror stories about the Japanese. On the train trip from Xian back to Zhengzhou and Wuhan, it was my good fortune to spend a day riding with the engineer in his wheezing, old steam locomotive. Mr. Li thought it would be good for me to experience firsthand the harassment the engineers were getting from the soldiers. And I figured the engineer might provide additional fodder for my exposé.

The heat from the firebox was almost unbearable. And so was the shriek of steam escaping from its leaky cylinders. But, fortunately, the engineer was a missionary school graduate from Nanjing and spoke enough English for us to carry on a limited conversation. He described how in 1937, the Japanese battered their way through the walls of Nanjing only to discover that Chiang Kai-shek and his government had escaped up the Yangtze River to Wuhan. Enraged that Chiang had eluded their grasp, the Japanese went on a looting, shooting, and raping rampage that left thousands of civilians stacked up dead in the street. *"Bu hao! Bu hao!"* ("Very bad! Very bad!"), exclaimed the engineer, assuming that I understood that much Chinese. Both his parents, he related, wiping away what was either a tear or drop of sweat, had been killed during the wholesale slaughter. Of course, the "Rape of Nanking," as it became known around the world, was considered one of the most savage assaults on civilians in the history of modern warfare. UNRRA officials in Washington had admitted during our indoctrination that the international wave of sympathy set off by that single catastrophic event was a major factor in establishing the relief program in China.

From Wuhan, the option existed to either fly back to Shanghai, a three-hour plane ride, or make the tortuous three-day trip by train. But boarding a plane in China back then was as risky as playing Russian roulette. Even so, I usually took the chance, or did until "Black Wednesday," as Christmas Day 1946 became known. The fog was so thick that eight of eleven flights scheduled to land in Shanghai were turned away, though the pilots claimed, "You can always get into Shanghai. It's flatter than piss on a platter." Nevertheless, the other three planes missed their approach and crashed into the nearby rice paddies, killing all sixty-seven passengers and their crews. The problem wasn't the terrain, but a lack of instrument training.

As it happened, I wouldn't have been aboard one those ill-fated planes anyway because on Christmas Day my Canadian roommate, Frank Boyer, was throwing a cocktail party for about a hundred of our UNRRA and CNRRA friends. Actually, it was a combination Christmas celebration, birthday party for Frank, and send-off for me, as I had just been ordered by Mr. Li to leave on a hazardous six-week-long round-trip by LST (Landing Ship Tank) to the Communist-held port of Yentai, or Chefoo, as it was then called. The CNRRA port officials there, Mr. Li explained, were being criticized in Washington for holding back the relief supplies earmarked for the Communists. My assignment was to try to break the bottleneck. Or, as I suspected, make it appear that CNRRA was sincere in trying to break the bottleneck. Part of the problem was the failure of the supplies to ever reach

Yentai. Nationalist air force fighters had strafed a couple of CNRRA supply ships headed there to discourage others from coming. Mr. Li knew this. But he decided to send me anyway, perhaps hoping I would refuse to go and resign, or worse.

Frank and I had recently moved into a cavernous, cream and gold tenth-floor suite in the Park Hotel, the perfect place for a party. This sleek, modern building overlooked the race course in the center of Shanghai. By the time Frank's party was over, fifteen trays of hors d'oeuvres prepared by Millie and her girlfriends, forty quarts of eggnog, and a case of Canadian Club whiskey had been consumed, leaving me hung over but happy to forsake the social rigors of Shanghai for the rugged voyage to Yentai.

The party was a huge success except for a couple of high-spirited guests who spied the dozens of quacking ducks crowded onto the third-floor terrace seven stories below our suite. The ducks were living out their last days before being baked crisp in the hotel's Chinese restaurant. Dangling hors d'oeuvres on long pieces of string as bait, the two inebriated guests engaged in a noisy contest to see who could lift one of the clipped-wing ducks highest in the air before it finally opened its beak, released the hors d'oeuvre, and crash-landed back on the terrace.

Frank and I had occasionally played this game ourselves without being apprehended. But this time the hotel manager stormed into the party. The next day he sent an eviction notice to the UNRRA billeting officer, who, fortunately for us, had been one of the avid duck baiters. When I returned from Yentai, all my belongings had been moved into the Cathay Hotel. The billeting officer felt so guilty about getting us thrown out of our hotel, he had relocated us in the swankiest one in all Shanghai. British-accented Chinese concierges in cutaways and striped pants manned the reception desk, while a swarm of young boy bellhops wearing starched white uniforms and white pillbox hats provided instant room service.

This elegant art deco structure facing the bund had a fascinating history. It was built by Sir Victor Sassoon, a local bon vivant whose Iraqi–Jewish forebears served as bankers to Baghdad's caliphs. Over the years it had become the meeting place for movie stars, writers, and diplomats. General George Marshall, sent by President Truman to China with the hopeless task of trying to convince Mao and Chiang to form a coalition government, stayed there. So did *New Yorker* correspondent Emily Hahn, with her pet gibbon, Mr. Mills, perched on her shoulder, and playwright Noel Coward, who spent several days nursing the flu and writing *Private Lives* in a suite that was subsequently named after him. Obviously, the Cathay was not the kind of place you would have expected UNRRA to pick for one of its billets. It was a whole world removed from the bawdy old "Greastern," where the relief agency first put its new recruits.

But those fancy Cathay digs were too luxurious to last. A few weeks later, we were transferred to the New Asia Hotel, a bare-bones billet overlooking the Suzhou Creek, in which most of the bathrooms were a fair hike down the hall. That last hotel switch had one advantage. Millie and her Canadian friend, Emilee Grant, shared a room there. But Frank and I had barely moved in when Mr. Li asked me to return to Yentai. The military situation there, and on the whole Shandong Peninsula, had deteriorated so that CNRRA was encountering even more trouble unloading its cargoes. Once again, my assignment was to try and break the bottleneck—at the risk of my own neck, though that didn't seem to worry Mr. Li, who had tired of my complaints about the squeeze being demanded by his operatives at every link of the CNRRA supply chain.

In March, while I was still in Yentai, the military situation became downright dangerous, making it impossible to carry out the assignment. The latest action centered around the mouth of the Yellow River (Huang Ho), where it empties into the Gulf of Bo Hai. As the *Wan Ching,* an LST carrying CNRRA supplies destined for the Communists, arrived in the gulf, a Nationalist plane plunked two bombs in the water beside it. Nobody was hurt, and the pilots apologized for their mistake. But shortly after that, when it and another LST, the *Wan Sze,* were discharging their supplies, Nationalist planes roared in for a repeat performance, raking the two CNRRA vessels from bow to stern with machine gun fire. One member of the Chinese crew was killed, two more were injured, a barge was sunk, and most of the cargo was destroyed. Great stuff for my exposé, but not for the destitute peasants in dire need of those relief supplies.

This time the Nationalist Army chief of staff, General Chen Cheng, sent a written apology to Harlan Cleveland, chief of the UNRRA mission in China. He promised there would be "no recurrence of these unfortunate accidents," which he attributed to "misidentification." But there was no mistaking the former U.S. Navy landing crafts for Communist vessels. Stripped of their antiaircraft guns, the LSTs displayed large UNRRA and CNRRA flags painted on their port and starboard sides.

Mao's propagandists played up the bombings as "more Nationalist outrages against the people of North China." But the Communists were hardly blameless. While the LSTs were being unloaded, they treated the crews to elaborate feasts. Brandy was plentiful in Shandong, and it flowed freely at these parties. Warmed by this unusual display of Communist hospitality, the crew members were then propositioned to smuggle guns and ammunition on future voyages.

During one banquet, it was also rumored that the skipper of the LST *Ching Ling,* sold the Communists his reserve fuel supply, pumping it ashore while the festivities were in full sway. But then finding trustworthy skippers in China was almost impossible. Most of the LST officers hired by CNRRA were either unlicensed or derelicts plucked off the beach in Shanghai.

These shenanigans finally came to a halt after yet another LST, the *Wan Shen,* was bombed and strafed by Nationalist P-47s. The bombs missed, but the planes darted back and forth over the hapless vessel, stitching her down the middle and riddling the bridge with bullets. Both the British captain and Canadian first officer were wounded and had to be evacuated by an American destroyer summoned to the scene. From his hospital bed in Shanghai, the wounded captain confessed that on the *Wan Shen*'s previous voyage some one hundred unmanifested cases labeled "hardware," had actually contained thirty-caliber ammunition. How much more contraband was smuggled to the Communists on these ships was never revealed.

After that futile attempt to break the bottleneck in the Bohai Gulf, my stay in Shanghai was short-lived. Mr. Li finally took the bull (me) by the horns and "promoted" me to chief transportation officer in Henan Province, a permanent assignment six hundred miles away from his CNRRA office, and from Millie.

3

CONVOYS TO NO-MAN'S LAND

Having visited Kaifeng on several previous trips to the interior I was surprised to find it preparing for war. Hundreds of Nationalist soldiers stood
guard at the massive iron gates and atop the city wall. Thousands more
roamed the muddy streets, flaunting their authority to conceal their war jit-
ters. Pillboxes had already been erected at the main intersections to defend
against street-by-street fighting. And, although it made no sense at all, an
occasional air raid drill was sprung on the hapless citizenry, who knew the
Communists had no warplanes. With sirens blaring and Nationalist Air
Force fighter planes droning overhead, the soldiers would thrust their bayonets at the disoriented crowds, kick over wheelbarrows left in their way,
and send the entire population scurrying for cover. When it was over, the
people would shrug their shoulders and go about their business of buying
and selling, sleeping and eating, procreating and dying.

During the Song Dynasty nine hundred years ago, Henan was known as
the Middle Province of the Middle Kingdom. Kaifeng then served as the
capital of all China, and not just of Henan. Historians also know it as the place
where large numbers of Jews traveling the old Silk Road finally settled, the
emperor having encouraged them to stay and "preserve the customs of your
ancestors." But the Jews were gradually assimilated and lost their identity.

Although the city was then called Xiangfu, meaning "fortunate sign," it was obvious when UNRRA picked Kaifeng for its regional headquarters that the signs were far from fortuitous. Floods, famine, and war had left the local populace crying for help. Foreign missionaries had done their best to relieve their misery, but the problems were just too immense.

Twenty-six times in Henan's history, the surging, silted Yellow River had wantonly changed course, flooding the towns below it. Known for centuries as "China's Sorrow" or the "Curse of the Sons of Han," the *Huang Ho* (Yellow River) was one of two monster dragons, alternately benevolent and merciless, that writhed completely across China. The other was the Yangtze, or Long Dragon River.

This century, just when the army of coolies manning the Yellow River dikes found they could keep pace with the silting process that constantly raised the riverbed and produced the floods, Chiang Kai-shek had seized on the Yellow River as a tactical weapon. Employing a "scorched earth" policy to try to stop the Japanese invaders in 1938, the generalissimo blew the dikes fifteen miles north of Zhengzhou. Some 890,000 of his countrymen perished. And as the alluvium spread south over the Central Plain, many more millions were made homeless.

Again, in 1946, Chiang decided to use the river as a weapon, this time in an attempt to seal off the armies of Mao Zedong in the north. Enlisting 50,000 wheelbarrow men, he changed the river's course back into its old bed. The feat was actually performed by the imperious UNRRA engineer O. J. Todd, known as "Todd Almighty," because of his arrogance, as well as for the miracle he performed in sealing the mile-long breach in the dike. As it turned out, Chiang's tactic didn't work any better against the Communists than it did against the Japanese. Mao's forces quickly ferried themselves across the river.

To rescue the vast populations affected by the river's altered course, UNRRA, in collaboration with CNRRA, launched two ambitious relief programs. The first, called the Yellow River Resettlement Program, was designed to relocate the 600,000 displaced peasants who eight years earlier had moved into the dried-up old bed, only to be chased out again by the returning waters.

The second, called the Flooded Area Program, which I had just been assigned to, was established to assist half a million other farmers and their families reclaim their land, which had been underwater before the gap closure project was completed. Although the five-thousand-square-mile area was slowly drying up, it continued to be called the "Flooded Area." Many of its former farmers feared that the land would once again be inundated and were reluctant to return. Only after UNRRA promised to provide them with the essentials for resettlement did they begin to come back.

To accomplish my mission as the newly arrived regional transportation chief, CNRRA handed me four hundred World War II trucks and seven hundred Chinese drivers and mechanics to run them. My army experience had been with DUKWs, not trucks. But Mr. Li, six hundred miles away in Shanghai, didn't seem to know the difference. Claude Lievsay, a young mechanical engineer from Ventura, California, had already been put in charge of maintenance. Together we were charged—according to the bureaucratic language of our CNRRA orders—with "organizing, implementing, and carrying out a supply operation that will provide the resettled families in the former flooded area south of Kaifeng with food, clothing, farm tools, seeds, and fertilizer."

I had read how recurring floods and famines had wiped out vast segments of the population in this part of the Central Plain. Theodore White's gruesome description of the 1943 famine there was the first thing that came to mind when I received my marching orders to head for Henan. It occurred to me that White's horrifying eyewitness account of a whole province practically dehumanized by mass starvation probably had a lot to do with the establishment of our relief program in Kaifeng.

"People fled the impersonal cruelty of hunger as if a barbarian army were upon them," White had written in *Thunder Out of China,* a book Chiang Kai-shek tried hard to suppress. "There were corpses on the road. A girl, slim and pretty, lay on the damp earth, her lips blue with death; her eyes were open and the rain fell on them. Men chipped at bark and pounded it by the roadside for food. A dog digging at a mound was exposing a human body."

According to White, the desperate, starving populace finally resorted to cannibalism. A doctor told him of a woman caught boiling her baby. Another woman, he claimed, had been found cutting off the legs of her dead husband for meat, while a number of refugees fleeing the area had been intercepted and killed for their flesh.

The people of Henan were no longer in such desperate straits when I arrived there in July 1947. Yet the recently flooded farmland, already mostly bone dry and barren, was being contested by Nationalist and Communist soldiers, who if not yet fighting for complete control, were at least stalking and taking potshots at each other, preparing for a showdown battle.

A hit-and-run vanguard 20,000 strong, commanded by General Zhang Xaohua, kept pinning down Nationalist units here and there, while elements of the Eighth Route Army, or *Ba Lu,* commanded by the "One-Eyed Dragon," General Liu Bocheng, probed all the way south to the Yangtze. A former cow herder, miner, and highway robber, the ruthless Liu was the most feared Communist general in all China. Also dropping into the area now and then was Mao's political emissary, Zhou Enlai, having been given the rank of brigadier general.

At the same time, making things difficult for our relief operations, General Chen Yi's Third Route Army, had peeled away 140 miles of Lunghai track, cutting the rail connection with Shanghai. Every time the Nationalists rebuilt the trestles, replaced the wood ties, and re-laid the old steel rails, the Communists would tear them up again. Because the rail service had become so unreliable, all of the spare parts for our trucks were being flown into Kaifeng by CAT, as General Claire Chennault's Civil Air Transport was called. The famous World War II Flying Tigers' commander had recruited many of his former P-40 fighter pilots to fly a fleet of war-surplus C-46 and C-47 transports in China.

The pilots were a colorful, swashbuckling bunch—heroes like Joe Rosbert, a Flying Tiger ace who had shot down seven Japanese Zeros; Lew Burridge; "Bus" Loane; and the black-bearded James McGovern, known as "Earthquake Magoon." Earthquake, whose airline pilot's uniform consisted of combat boots and a T-shirt inflated by a huge beer belly, became a legend in China after Milton Caniff, the creator of *Terry and the Pirates,* turned him into a comic strip character.

Most of the time, the old planes with a newborn tiger kitten painted on their nose, were chartered by the Nationalists to fly guns and ammunition to isolated army units or to rescue civilians fleeing the Communists. So UNRRA had to settle for second call on the planes. But once a week a fat-bellied C-46 laden with spare parts for our trucks would land in Kaifeng. It was our main contact with the outside world. The pilots could be counted on to bring our mail and newspapers, and always a fresh batch of rumors about the shifting tides of the civil war.

It was under these challenging conditions that Claude Lievsay and I plunged into our new assignment, naively hoping that the immunity promised by the two warring sides would allow us to carry out our mission unmolested. But the chances of our eventually getting sucked into the civil war seemed inevitable. There were just too many soldiers and weapons around.

Right from the beginning, we discovered that either Claude or I, or both of us together, had to escort the truck convoys if they were to reach their destinations without being looted by either Nationalist or Communist soldiers. Sometimes it was hard to tell which army the looters belonged to because the war front was so fluid that many of the mud-walled towns and villages changed hands every week or two. The roads were a worse problem. Never intended for motor vehicles, they had been worn into existence by a 2,000-year procession of ox carts, mule carts, and wheelbarrows. Even the so-called highways were merely deep grooves ground into the sun-baked loess and covered over by a six-inch blanket of silky red dust.

Bumping along at the head of the convoy, I would gingerly ease my jeep in and out of craters and over humps. But after a few weeks, patience and care gave way to sheer masochism. I started stomping the accelerator, smashing into holes, or taking off into the air. The windshield might crack, the springs might snap, and the radiator needed re-soldering after almost every trip. Still, the engine kept whining angrily as I sucked in mouthfuls of red dust. Lurking in the back of my mind was the hope that with the next solid whack my battered jeep might lie down and die. Then I could walk, as was intended, on these ancient highways.

Following my jeep, banging along at a fifteen-mile-an-hour clip, were thirty or forty trucks, a mongrel convoy composed of former U.S. Army and Navy ten-wheel GMCs and Internationals, smaller civilian Dodges, Studebakers, Chevys, and Fords. A couple of ugly, blunt-nosed Canadian Fords always took up the rear. "Yellow fish," as the illegal passengers were called, perched dangerously atop many of the tarpalulin-covered loads.

The runs our trucks made were considered routine because CNRRA convoys laden with sacks of American flour and rice, or bales of old clothing, repeated the trips every few days. But from my standpoint, no convoy starting out in Nationalist territory and threading its way across a bleak no-man's-land into Communist territory could be considered routine. To keep our trucks from being shot at, CNRRA had painted them with yellow and black tiger stripes. Still, the clean bullet hole in a corner of my jeep's windshield served as a constant reminder that a mere paint job offered little protection.

The shooting began when Claude and I were jouncing along mindlessly. Three bullets slammed into our jeep. One bullet glanced off the hood, another punctured the left rear tire, and the third just missed Claude's head before piercing the windshield. We never found out who was trying to kill us, or why. Probably Nationalists pretending to be Communists, we concluded. However, the Chinese drivers of the trucks trailing behind needed no bullet holes in their vehicles to remind them that a war was going on. They had a way of melting into the countryside at the first sound of gunfire, leaving the convoy stalled.

That close call made Claude wonder whether he was ever again going to see Lilly, the young Eurasian girl in Shanghai whom he was engaged to marry. He had already picked me for his best man. "The wedding can take place without you," he joked. "But I'm essential."

I, too, worried that a better-aimed bullet could end what had turned into a long-distance romance with Millie. But a week later I was stunned to see her step off a supply plane in Kaifeng, having wangled a transfer to UNRRA's Henan Province headquarters. Millie was a wangler all right. She wasn't artful. But I was sure the unsophisticated country-girl grin rendered her bosses defenseless, unable to refuse her requests, even one that meant losing her services. She once told me how she'd gotten herself transferred from one government job to another all the way from tiny Saint Regis Falls, New York, where she grew up, down to the nation's capital and the job with UNRRA.

Her latest transfer solved my loneliness problem, but not the difficulty to getting the relief supplies into the hands of those desperately needing them. Further complicating that job was an edict from Washington, D.C. issued by Fiorello LaGuardia, the former mayor of New York City, who now headed UNRRA. He stipulated that 30 percent of all relief supplies shipped to China were to be distributed in Communist-held areas, the rest of it in Nationalist territory. Fair enough in theory. But in practice it was impossible to divvy up the food, clothing, fertilizer, farm tools, and other supplies that precisely, just as it was impossible to jeep across the rough terrain without painfully jouncing your innards.

The ninety-mile trip from Kaifeng to Xihua was the most frequent one made by our convoys—our milk run so to speak. With luck, the trucks could cover the distance in nine hours. Without luck, it might take them several days. If the convoy got bogged down by the war, weather, or mechanical failures, the trucks would pull in behind the protective walls of a town. But the small population centers of Henan had no hotels or even government guesthouses, so the drivers would head for the local whorehouse—not for sex, just to sleep. Squatting on the dirt floor, they'd while away the evening sipping tea, chewing watermelon seeds, and chatting with the girls before rolling up in the blankets they brought with them.

If there was a Jesuit mission in town, I would usually stay there, both for sanitary and social reasons. As in Bengpu, the fathers and brothers in Henan were always grateful for a Western visitor. But if there was no mission then I, too, would be stuck with the whores, though their nightlong nattering made it difficult to sleep.

Xuchang, a Nationalist stronghold located between Kaifeng and Xihua, was our main storage and distribution center. We frequently encountered long files of Chiang Kai-shek's soldiers marching through its streets. They appeared to be trim fighting units armed with tommy-guns and light and heavy machine guns and clad in new tan summer uniforms. Without fail, one of the officers would stop our convoy. The first time that happened, I thought he was out to commandeer one or two of our trucks, which was not an uncommon occurrence even though in addition to their distinctive yellow and black tiger stripes the trucks flew CNRRA flags from their right front fenders. The officer surely had seen our trucks many times before. But it gave him face to hold up the convoy before a gawking crowd of civilian bystanders while he peppered my interpreter with questions.

Where was the convoy headed? What does the cargo consist of? Who is it for? Soldiers brandishing tommy-guns would break ranks and cover the convoy menacingly during this grilling. It was a good show and, obviously, the civilian bystanders enjoyed it. But everyone knew the Nationalist soldiers only did this sort of bullying inside the city's high walls.

In an age that already knew the destructive power of an atomic bomb, it was hard to appreciate the protection afforded by a mud wall. In China, however, a city wall forty feet high and twenty or thirty feet thick was still considered a formidable defense against infantry attack. Hiding behind these ramparts gave the local commanders and their troops a sense of security.

Rarely did the Nationalist troops venture far outside, where they might encounter the enemy. In fact, there seemed to be a military understanding in Henan Province—the Nationalists could cling to the major cities and roadways, while the Communists infiltrated the farmland and hacked away at the rail lines. Only when the Communists attempted to capture a strategic city did a skirmish ensue. Then Chiang Kai-shek's soldiers were forced to come out from behind their protective walls, like foxes flushed out of their holes, and fight.

Xuchang, one of our distribution centers, I discovered was an ancient market place that got its name from Emperor Cao in A.D. 200. He called it the Kingdom of Xu. Chairman Mao, whose troops were now threatening to overrun the place, had renamed it the Kingdom of Tobacco because of its cigarette factories. By any name, Xuchang's strategic location fifty miles below China's key rail hub of Zhengzhou, made it a prime target. Mao had recently boasted that his armies were prepared to rip up the north-south Ping-Han rail line, as well as the east-west Lunghai line, thereby nailing the Nationalists to the Zhengzhou cross, the city where the two lines intersected. Rumors (*yao-yen*) flew that if that happened, Xuchang would fall like a ripe melon into Mao's hands.

The city's 200,000 residents needed no more rumors. In fact, spreading rumors there was a crime punishable by death. Even facts were considered rumors until they were officially revealed. But the people didn't have to speculate on how dangerous the situation was. The signs were obvious. Thousands of coolies, conscripted without pay, were out every day patching the thick forty-foot-high wall and widening the moat around it. All the gates except one were barricaded with huge timbers and strung with concertina rolls of barbed wire. At the open gate, a squad of Nationalist soldiers frisked all travelers, poking their bundles and baskets with bayonets. Few of the sentries could read, but they scrutinized every traveler's identity card with exaggerated care.

From Xuchang, our convoys had to cross the disputed no-man's-land to reach Communist-held Xihua. This was an area that both armies claimed, but neither controlled. Instead, they simply took turns taxing and looting the towns located in it. On the return trip from Xihua, it was not unusual to find that all the Nationalist sentries in the towns along the way had been replaced by Communist sentries, or vice versa. This changing of the guard often had been accomplished bloodlessly.

Once I asked a Nationalist sentry guarding the arched gate to the village of Wunudian what he would do if a Communist column came marching down the road. He didn't answer, and my interpreter later reprimanded me for being impolite. "Naturally, the sentry would run away," my interpreter explained.

Translated literally, Wunudian means "Five Girls Town." Legend had it that a retired warlord and his five daughters founded a thriving tea shop there some fifteen centuries ago. When it was discovered that the girls were peddling more than tea, they were run out of town. But the place remained a provincial landmark for all wayfarers, including our drivers.

It was clear that few changes had been wrought in Wunudian during the intervening millennium-and-a-half. As in most Henan villages, its main street was a deep, sandy hollow running from gate to gate. Centuries of through traffic had worn the narrow street down ten feet below the level of the mud houses on each side. Chickens, ducks, and pigs scooted out of the way of our oncoming convoys, trying to squeeze through, while a couple of mangy dogs would usually rouse themselves from sunbaths in the middle of the road and limp away. Most of the dogs in China appeared to be crippled. In the Communist areas even hale and hearty canines were exterminated, and in some cases eaten, because dog meat was considered a delicacy. The Communists, however, considered food too precious to waste on pets.

The whine of our trucks passing through Wunudian, or any other town for that matter, would drown out the shrieking and clapping of the kids racing excitedly beside them. They looked like miniature Buddhas, but with bare bottoms protruding from their split-tail rompers, a Chinese innovation eliminating the need for diapers. The village children were not accustomed to our big four-by-four trucks. Every week or so, a tot somewhere along our route would become frightened by the noise and swirling dust and try to scamper between the oncoming vehicles. Or, worse yet, dart underneath between the front and rear wheels.

According to what was then Chinese law, in all accidents involving a motor vehicle and a pedestrian, the driver was considered at fault. The law was simple enough, though sometimes its interpretation became difficult. During one of our runs, a soldier was killed by a CNRRA truck. The driver was summarily carted off to jail, only to be released when it was discovered that the soldier had hitched a ride and had accidentally fallen off the truck. Three days later, the driver was back in jail. It turned out the soldier had not really hitched a ride, but had forced the driver at gunpoint to pick him up. That made no difference because it was also confirmed that the soldier had fallen beneath the truck's wheels. Clearly, the driver had run over him. To avoid legal complications like that, CNRRA drivers were authorized to make a fifty-dollar roadside settlement with the victim's family in every fatal accident.

The next stretch of road between Wunudian and Yanling was pretty good, running through what resembled the flat wheat-growing land of Kansas. As a matter of fact, not too many years ago, Henan adopted Kansas as its sister state and entertained the American governor on a visit. But this road, even during the civil war days, was good enough so my jeep kept jouncing along at a thirty-mile-an-hour clip. With the windshield wipers ticking evenly back and forth and rivulets of dry dust streaming down the glass like rain, my thoughts tended to wander until they lit upon the one question that kept hounding me: "Why are you risking your rear end running a bunch of trucks through some other country's civil war?" What I really wanted to do was write. To bear witness to the people and events changing China.

My typewriter and camera were always tucked away in the jeep. Taking pictures posed no problem. It was easy to stop the convoy and crank off a few shots. And photo opportunities, like the ant-like processions of wheelbarrows passing by, presented themselves at almost every turn of the road. It was nothing for a man to push a five-hundred-pound wheelbarrow a hundred miles in a week. If he heard shooting up ahead, he'd stop and wait for it to subside, just as he did if rain washed out the road. Picturesque lines of women with heavy bundles suspended from *biandan* (shoulder poles) also trudged by, their loads jouncing rhythmically up and down. It was difficult to pass these wayfarers without aiming my Minoltaflex at them, although Chinese superstition against being photographed made many of my best subjects run away. The writing, however, came much harder. It was difficult to settle down at a typewriter after being hammered all day on one of China's rutted highways. My "UNRRA in Bandit Land" exposé was coming along so slowly I feared my agent in New York might have given up hope of getting it.

On clear days, the high mud wall of Yanling, the next town on our route across the barren no-man's-land, was visible from a mile away. The main gate was always locked and barricaded, preventing our trucks from passing through. Crudely painted Chinese characters above the sealed entryway exhorted passersby to SUPPORT GENERALISSIMO CHIANG KAI-SHEK'S MOBILIZATION ORDER AND FIGHT THE COMMUNIST BANDITS. A poster tacked to the gate, which I stopped the convoy to photograph, pictured a Chinese fist knocking Mao out of China, while Yen Wang, the king of hell, beckoned to him with death's claw.

Fortunately, there was no need to harangue the guards to open the gate and let our convoy through. A freshly hacked-out detour skirted the city along its moat. A small creek emptied into the moat. I liked to park beside it and watch the fishermen skillfully dipping their nets into the creek and then swiftly raising them up again. Occasionally, a tiny, silvery minnow wriggled in the cloudy red water as a net broke the surface.

The easiest thing to obtain in China was an audience. A crowd of old geezers soaking up the sun on a stone bridge was always there, watching the fishermen. And a couple of young boys would often scramble up from under the bridge to inspect my jeep—and, of course, me. Most of the time I traveled shirtless, and the boys could never resist rubbing the hair on my chest—a rarity on the chests of Chinese men—to see if it was real. Once I responded by tousling a boy's head and kidding him in Chinese.

"You're my good friend," I said, whereupon his father suddenly appeared and asked if I wanted to take the boy with me. In rapid Chinese, not all of which I understood, the father explained that he had six other children and not enough food for all of them. It would be much better for the boy if I adopted him. His grin was seductive and, for a fleeting moment, I thought of bringing the boy back to our headquarters in Kaifeng and making him a mascot for our trucking operation. He could have run errands around the compound. But once UNRRA completed its mission, he would have become homeless and worse off than he was in Yanling.

After skirting Yanling, our convoys entered the part of the no-man's-land still known as the Flooded Area, although the ground in most paces was bone-dry. At this point I would switch to the rear of the convoy to prod the stragglers, trying to keep those tail-end trucks from being picked off by either Nationalist or Communist soldiers. The Nationalists were the real culprits. They had a nasty habit of grabbing two or three trucks at a time, stealing the cargo, and then turning them into troop carriers until they ran out of gas and had to be abandoned.

Our convoys were especially vulnerable on this leg of the journey. Most of the remaining water in the Flooded Area consisted of shallow pools easy for our trucks to ford. But there were still a few deepwater crossings that the trucks had to be rafted across one at a time, making them sitting ducks for a band of marauding soldiers. We begged UNRRA to assign security guards to these crossings. But our pleas went unanswered.

Curly Chu, my interpreter, who usually rode "shotgun" in a truck at the tail end of the convoy, would take my place at the head of the convoy on this part of the trip. Fukou, the next town, was usually occupied by the Communists. Curly knew a couple of their officers, and he could always find out quickly if they were going to give us any trouble.

It may have been Curly's fluent English or his tall, strong build, or perhaps it was his curly hair, but I never thought of him as being Chinese. Only twenty-two, he had acquired many American mannerisms working for CNRRA, including a consuming passion for pretty Western women. And there were a couple of pretty ones besides Millie assigned to the UNRRA office in Kaifeng. "A Shandong man is like a thermos bottle," Curly once told me, "cold on the outside, but hot on the inside." However, Curly's ardor hadn't stopped him from leaving his Chinese girlfriend behind in Shandong when he signed on with CNRRA. Even stronger, I suspected, was his desire for a visa to the U.S., which he hoped to obtain through his newfound American contacts.

The sandy wasteland slowly gave way to cultivated furrows flanking the highway as our convoys rolled south. Newly built farming villages dotted the landscape. Each village consisted of a collection of crude one-room structures. They were built out of dried sorghum stalks, the *gaoliang* from which the Chinese brewed *bai-gar,* the throat-scorching white lightning that did me in during those unavoidable bottoms-up toasts.

On one trip through this area, Curly led me inside a few farmhouses to show me what they were like. "These people live very simply," he warned. But that was an understatement. The square mud huts with thatched roofs made of dried sorghum were almost identical. So were the interiors. A straw bed occupied more than half the floor space. In one corner, an iron pot rested on a brick stove. There was one porcelain bowl and a pair of chopsticks for each family member. A small mound of beans and a few dried bones constituted the customary larder. Most of the time, all of the clothes a family owned were worn to work in and sleep in, as well. But their poverty didn't stop the occupants from smiling as Curly rattled off an explanation of what this inquisitive American was doing in Henan Province. "Does it rain where you come from?" one of them inquired, the same question a peasant had asked when I was bicycling around Bengpu with Father Minella. Evidently, some Chinese farmers wondered if rain might be a special gift from heaven bestowed only on China.

Although the reclaimed farmland was being fiercely contested by both Nationalists and Communists, the farmers and their families seemed unpersuaded by the propaganda barrage from either side. "If you're a soldier," one of the farmers explained to Curly, "you must fight with one army or the other. If you're a magistrate you must be a Nationalist magistrate or a Communist magistrate. But if you're a farmer, that's what you are."

In an American magazine I had read about a nonpolitical farmer like this one, whose land had been overrun from time to time, first by first Nationalists and then by Communists. "Which side is better?" he was asked. "They're both good," the peasant answered tactfully. "Only the people are bad."

In Fukou, as far as I was concerned, the people always behaved badly. The first time the Communists occupied the town, they published a roster of the richest families whose houses could be ransacked by all comers in an informal wealth equalization plan. Only removable items, it was expected, would be taken. But after hundreds of spirited looters had cleaned out all the dinnerware, furniture, and other valuables, they took to unhinging the doors, prying out the window frames, and peeling wood panels from the walls. When a few latecomers arrived and started chipping out bricks and removing roof tiles, they were hauled off to the dike and shot.

Four days later, the Nationalists returned. Since when had looting been legalized? they asked. An order was issued to immediately return all the stolen items. And to make certain everybody took the order seriously, a dozen more of the worst offenders were taken out to the same dike and shot through the head. But the Nationalist authorities failed to mention where the loot was to be returned. When the sun came up the next morning, all the stolen stuff was scattered in the streets.

Fukou was one of the few cities in the region that had been severely damaged during the fighting. Hit first by Communist artillery shells and then by Nationalist dive-bombers, a gaping hole had been blown in the outer wall, and several of the buildings inside had been shorn of their roofs or completely gutted. But as was true in many of the neighboring towns, the sudden policy reversals implemented every time the city changed hands caused as much havoc as the fighting.

We could always tell whether Fukou was in Communist or Nationalist hands by the sentry silhouetted against the sun standing atop the high wall. If the Nationalists were in control, our drivers usually stopped there for lunch. Otherwise, the convoy would roll right on through, forcing the curbside food vendors to hastily pull in their rickety stands so the trucks could squeeze by.

In what was still unoccupied wasteland south of Fukou, we often encountered the same Nationalist and Communist battalions tracking each other across the plain, but always about ten miles apart in what appeared to be a mock war. They never clashed. The Nationalist troops were smartly dressed, their machine guns glinting in the afternoon sun, as they trudged along on foot. Their commanding officer, mounted on a black pony, would always canter over to watch our convoy pass. For officers like him, the army could be a profitable business. As the reigning local authority, he was free to shake down the wealthy merchants in the nearby towns and villages, or even sell some of his battalion's artillery pieces and other weapons to the enemy. For his lowly foot soldiers, the army was at least a meal ticket. But from battalion commander down to private there was little will to fight.

The Communists were a ragtag bunch, but had the reputation for being fierce fighters when called into battle. This particular battalion wore peasant garb, and in some of their squads no two rifles appeared to match. But at that stage of the civil war, Mao's soldiers relied mainly on old muskets and rarely carried more than four or five rounds of ammunition. Sometimes they were even forced to skimp on the powder charge in their bullets. I once encountered a Nationalist private who'd been shot in the neck, but the bullet had bounced off, leaving only a bad bruise. The best weapons the Communists possessed were those captured or purchased from the Nationalists.

Although the Communist military strategy was carefully planned, coordination between units in the field appeared to be amazingly loose. Once we encountered Communist sentries guarding a town, unaware that an entire Red division was camped a few miles down the road. Another time, a Communist battalion attacked Fukou only to discover it was trying to take the city from a Red battalion that had captured it the day before.

Driving further into the Flooded Area, our trucks ran through deep Sahara-like sand, signaling the approach of Xihua. Even in four-wheel drive, my jeep labored hard to keep its forward momentum. When the tires gripped solid ground it sped ahead for a few yards, then slowed almost to a full stop as the wheels spun freely in the sand. It was also easy to tell when we were approaching Xihua by the whine of the trucks pushing from behind. Instinctively, the drivers speeded up when they entered what they considered were the badlands of Communist territory—not that the Communist soldiers were any more menacing than the Nationalists, but anti-Communist posters placed near our truck terminal in Kaifeng depicted bayonettings and beheadings by the Reds in this part of Henan. The drivers recognized the posters as propaganda. Even so, the posters made a deep impression, especially those picturing human heads impaled on pungi sticks planted along the road—the same scare tactic used by the Communists in Vietnam.

Control of Xihua was no longer seesawing back and forth, as was the case in many of the towns our convoys supplied. For five months it had been firmly in Communist hands. Every time we went there the cadres of peasant militiamen camped outside the city wall seemed to be growing. Xihua, it appeared, was being used as a staging area for fighting elsewhere in Henan. Still, the young soldiers looked like farm boys except for their blue caps, and rifles slung muzzle-down across their backs. Unlike these ragtag trainees, the Communist sentries posted at the city gate sported new blue uniforms and polished rifles. They saluted smartly and, with a quick flick of their bayonets, motioned the convoy to pass.

Inside its high walls, Xihua resembled any other city in Henan, except for the anti-American posters picturing a gluttonous Uncle Sam biting big chunks from the heart of China. That message obviously eluded the kids who ran in swarms beside our trucks babbling greetings to the drivers and shouting *Meiguoren dinghao!* ("Americans very good") when they spotted my jeep.

The sight of an American bringing much-needed food and clothing to Xihua also contradicted what was being printed in the local Communist newspaper. Blaring headlines labeled UNRRA and CNRRA personnel as "aggressors in the name of relief." Editorial tirades accused "traitor Chiang" of allowing American relief representatives to travel freely throughout China, "collecting military secrets and surveying economic resources." Most of Xihua's citizens dismissed those charges as propaganda. Only when a Nationalist P-47 dropped an occasional bomb on them did the accusations hit home. Everyone knew the planes and bombs were made in America.

It was difficult to tell how the anti-American propaganda affected our drivers. In fact, it was often hard to tell on whose side the drivers were really on. They were well traveled, decently paid, and far more sophisticated than peasants working the land or shopkeepers stuck in small towns. Yet, they were an inscrutable bunch, believing it best to keep their mouths shut if they wanted to keep their jobs.

As the civil war intensified and tensions heightened, it occurred to me that a couple of our drivers might be Communist plants. After all, Mao had good reason to keep abreast of CNRRA's operations, knowing that the Nationalists were doing their best to keep our relief supplies from reaching his areas. Even so, I'd never seriously worried about our trucking operation being infiltrated. Then, one day, I spotted one of our drivers chatting with Xihua's Communist Party boss. I understood enough Chinese to catch the drift of their conversation. That was strange. A party boss chatting with a trucker? Then it hit me. From the party boss's respectful tone, the driver probably outranked him. I was stunned. Communist spies in our local CNRRA outfit was one problem I'd never reckoned with. But it was one, I realized, I would have to deal with from now on—especially if the number of Communist attacks on our convoys continued to grow.

4

CRISIS IN KAIFENG

By August 1947, the situation in Henan was disintegrating on all fronts. Nationalist military defenses were crumbling, precipitating a whirlwind visit by Chiang Kai-shek to bolster the sagging morale of his troops. At the same time, Communist complaints were becoming more shrill about the unfair distribution of relief supplies in the province, resulting in the unexpected appearance of Mao's personal envoy, Zhou Enlai. And UNRRA and CNRRA personnel in Kaifeng were suddenly demanding armed protection, forcing Harlan Cleveland, the relief agency's boss in Shanghai, to fly in and calm everybody down.

The generalissimo was the first to arrive. The day began like any other. A long line of men, women, children, oxen, mules, dogs, chickens, and pigs stood quietly outside Kaifeng's city wall. They were waiting for daybreak, when the soldiers normally opened the heavy, spiked iron gate so they could proceed inside to sell their goods. The Chinese are a patient people, and the war had made them more so. But on this particular morning they grumbled to the soldiers because the gate remained closed.

At the railroad station inside the city, the waiting scene was repeated. Streaks of light were beginning to show in the sky above the sea of weary travelers sprawled out on the platform beside their belongings. As they commenced to stir, young girls carrying kettles of warm water and cakes of soap in brass basins circulated through the crowd, charging five hundred Chinese dollars (one cent) a wash. But the rail yard behind the station stayed quiet except for the shouts of a few naked, soot-smeared children picking through the ashes for pieces of coal for their mothers to sell. The eastbound express arriving from Xian and proceeding on to Xuzhou, Nanjing, and Shanghai, hadn't appeared for two days. And it wouldn't again today, the stationmaster announced, though nobody knew why.

The city center, too, was just coming awake. The clock atop the thousand-year-old drum tower, where men once thumped out the hours on huge brass drums, struck six. That signaled the lifting of the all-night curfew, not that it was very carefully observed. Those people who had business to tend to after dark would walk through the ink-black streets listening for the click of a rifle bolt, or the cry, "Halt!" coming from an unseen sentry. But everyone knew the sentries had orders not to shoot.

At the sound of the drum tower clock, shopkeepers on *Sheng Fu Lu* (Provincial Government Street) began to peel the protective board panels from their display windows. The honey cart men were already out collecting the pungent human excrement for delivery to the outlying farms. A few rickshaw boys padded noiselessly up and down the street, pulling early-morning fares. Others stood in the shafts of their rickshaws slurping noodles from crockery bowls. An oxcart creaked by, the sharp crack of the driver's whip shattering the morning air.

A boy suddenly raced down the street chattering excitedly to the rickshaw boys and shopkeepers, "The soldiers are coming! The soldiers are coming!" Soon, soldiers swarmed down *Sheng Fu Lu* and the traffic stopped. Shopkeepers hurriedly put back the boards on their windows, while the pedestrians, rickshaws, carts, and animals were herded into the alleys and side streets.

Rumors flew. The One-Eyed Liu Bocheng and his Red Bandits were attacking from the north. General Chang Shao-hua had broken out of the Flooded Area and was attacking from the south. The dikes had burst and Kaifeng would soon be flooded.

Scare headlines, mobilization orders, and emergency proclamations were always accepted with stoic calm in Kaifeng. But when the gates remained shut, when the trains stopped running, when the people were herded off the streets and all work came to a halt, something truly bad must be happening. Then a strange sight dispelled everyone's worst fears. Platoons of coolies carrying shovels over their shoulders trudged down *Sheng Fu Lu*. They quickly dispersed and set to work leveling off the bumps and filling deep ruts and holes in the dirt street.

Amazing! The streets hadn't been repaired in years. Then more coolies with shovels arrived, and the tempo of the work increased. Soon, all the way down *Sheng Fu Lu* the clank and scrape of shovels could be heard as the coolies labored with unusual vigor.

The bamboo telegraph works fast in China, and a fresh rumor swept the city: The generalissimo is coming. What else could move the municipal authorities to repair *Sheng Fu Lu*?

This rumor caught hold. Shopkeepers quickly splashed whitewash over their storefronts and swept their walks. Women hurriedly dressed their children, ordinarily allowed to run naked through the streets. Overhead, the air suddenly droned with the sound of P-51 fighter planes circling the city.

An olive-colored C-47 hovered over Kaifeng, and then descended onto the concrete airstrip left by the Japanese. A few minutes later, a motorcade of armed trucks and dilapidated official cars roared down the freshly smoothed street. In the middle of this procession appeared a shiny black limousine, and as it sped by I glimpsed the baldheaded generalissimo sitting erect in the back seat.

The Minoltaflex was hanging from my neck, but the limo sped by too fast to grab the camera and knock off a shot. My next impulse was to whip off an eyewitness account of what was happening. The generalissimo's unexpected visit at this precarious moment in the war must be significant. Certainly, it was news. But why bother, I thought. There was no telegraph office in Kaifeng. And I had no contact with any wire service in Shanghai that might want an exclusive account. Nevertheless, my journalistic juices were flowing. The urge to report what was going on was hard to contain.

Watching the motorcade pull up at the provincial government head-quarters and Chiang disappear inside, I had to remind myself that this was no comic-opera character like the one cartooned by the Communist propagandists—a generalissimo weighted down by medals, lopping off Chinese heads with a long sword. Nor was this the "Peanut," as General "Vinegar Joe" Stilwell, the acerbic American World War II commander in China, had nicknamed him. No, this was one of the world's "Big Five," the leader who dared to challenge the anti-Japanese strategy of Winston Churchill and Franklin Roosevelt by arguing for an Allied invasion of China from the sea.

I had read about their summit meeting in Cairo, at which the American president and British prime minister finally placated the stubborn generalissimo by promising to give China all of the territory it had lost during its half-century struggle with Japan. Still vivid in my mind was the famous photograph of the leaders sitting side-by-side in front of the Nile: Chiang posing confidently in his crisply pressed uniform; next to him the crippled FDR; then Sir Winston in a rumpled white suit with a gray homburg resting on his lap. On the extreme right, chic as ever in a Chinese gown that looked like it came from Bergdorf Goodman in New York, sat the smiling Madame Chiang. Now, here in the flesh, was Chiang Kai-shek, without a reporter within six hundred miles to record this historic moment.

Suddenly, I envisioned myself conducting a Q & A with the generalissimo. My imagination had catapulted me into the back seat of that black limo, where I was peppering him with questions.

"Mr. President, how can your armies keep control of the Central Plain when your generals are selling their weapons to the enemy?" Good question, but unnecessarily insulting. Better be polite. The generalissimo is known for his temper. Just about every American in China had heard the apocryphal story of how in a fit of rage he'd shot his wife's dog.

"Mr. President, do you expect more American military aid?" I knew Truman feared becoming bogged down in China's civil war. Yet there was a powerful lobby at work in Washington agitating for more help for Chiang. And I suspected the generalissimo was counting heavily on it.

"Mr. President, many Americans consider Mao and his followers to be agrarian reformers, not hard-line Communists. Do you agree? And if so, is there any chance of you and Mao sharing power in a coalition government?" That, I realized, was a loaded question, or rather two loaded questions. First off, Chiang didn't care whether or not Mao was a dyed-in-the-wool Communist. He was the enemy. And, second, despite General George Marshall's best efforts to convince them to form a coalition, all the Nationalist newspapers predicted Mao and Chiang would never join forces.

Before my imaginary interview was over, the motorcade had pulled up at the provincial government headquarters. The generalissimo quickly disappeared inside, and a cordon of guards sprang into position around the building.

For five hours Kaifeng hung in suspense. The fighter planes kept on droning overhead, but on the street the soldiers relaxed their vigil, permitting the people to come out. They crept cautiously from the shops and houses to gape at the array of vehicles parked at the end of *Sheng Fu Lu*. Mothers nudged their children, pointing to the well-guarded provincial headquarters, while the men speculated on the reasons for the generalissimo's visit. On one thing they agreed—it was a bad sign. Chiang was probably there to prod his generals to stand and fight, which everyone knew they were reluctant to do.

At 3:00 P.M., the guards surrounding the government headquarters sprang to attention again. The soldiers posted in the street sent the crowds scurrying inside. The armed trucks and cars, including the shiny black limo, sped back up *Sheng Fu Lu*. Once again, I caught a fleeting glimpse of the erect figure propped up in the back seat. Then, as suddenly as he had come, the generalissimo was gone.

What intrigued me most about this man was the way he had dominated China for twenty years, yet remained an enigma to Americans. General Stilwell was outraged by Chiang's military ineptness. He couldn't understand why this convert to Christianity would preach Confucianism to his troops, or waste men and ammunition trying to contain the Communists before the Japanese were defeated. But could the "Peanut," have played off one warlord against another, or won the backing of China's bankers, traditionally distrustful of the military? No, and neither could a mere peanut move vast armies, evacuate whole cities, or, for that matter, procure the engineering services of UNRRA to change the course of a mighty river. A tyrant, perhaps, could do all of those things. Not a peanut.

Glimpsing this controversial Nationalist leader once again triggered my yearnings to bear witness, to decipher confusing world figures, and to analyze the intangible chemistry of their power. Men like Chiang, whose skill or skullduggery, jugular timing, and, above all, ability to make things happen, had always fascinated me. Ordinary people might be more appealing, but they didn't preoccupy my thoughts in the same way. No matter how bleak the job prospects in journalism, the time was fast approaching to quit CNRRA and pursue a reporting career.

The frustration of not being able to tell the story of Chiang's unexpected visit prompted my application to the Columbia University Graduate School of Journalism—with the added hope, as a war veteran, of going there on the G.I. Bill. It was very late to be applying for the fall semester, and my grades at Dartmouth had only been fair. But my energies at college had been focused on getting campus scoops for the *Boston Post* and the *Springfield Republican,* not on academics. The admissions people at Columbia, I figured, would appreciate that, as well as my time spent in the merchant marine and army, followed by more than a year in China.

A week after Chiang's whirlwind visit, what could have been another journalistic coup fell into my lap. Without warning, the UNRRA headquarters in Kaifeng found itself playing host to Brigadier General Zhou Enlai, Mao's political troubleshooter, who one day would become China's premier. Unlike the generalissimo, he slipped into town unnoticed. His message to UNRRA was blunt. Mao, he reported, was infuriated by our failure to deliver the apportioned relief supplies to the "liberated areas," the Communist term for the parts of China under their control. Had one of my spying CNRRA drivers contacted Zhou? That was my first thought, though it turned out Zhou was simply citing LaGuardia's decree earmarking 30 percent of the relief supplies for the Communists. To make certain they got their fair share, Mao had established CLARA, the acronym for Communist Liberated Area Relief Association. But ever since the Nationalists began bombing and strafing CNRRA's supply ships while they were unloading in Yentai—the Shandong port where Mr. Li had sent me on those wild goose chases—the flow of food, clothing, and agricultural equipment destined for the Communists had been reduced to a trickle. "You must stand up for us," Zhou insisted, adding words to the effect that he and Mao considered UNRRA and CNRRA personnel a bunch of weak-kneed bureaucrats for caving in to the Nationalists.

After his tough head-to-head session with the UNRRA boss in Kaifeng, Zhou softened up and agreed to spend the night at our compound. Our offices and living quarters were divided between two identical Western-style brick residences that the Chinese had dubbed *Hong Anlu* (red-gabled buildings). A spare bedroom was given to Zhou. Although he spoke spotty English, learned in an American missionary school in Tianjin (Tientsin), as well as French and German, picked up during his student days in Paris and Berlin, he spoke to us in Chinese using one of our interpreters to translate.

Unlike Chiang and Mao, both of them peasants risen to power, Zhou was the son of a well-to-do mandarin. I was surprised during dinner how urbane and witty the man was. Lively dark eyes peered out from under heavy eyebrows that looked like they'd been pasted on. When he smiled, which he did frequently, long vertical furrows creased his cheeks. A scraggly beard adorned his chin, though I'd heard he frequently shaved it off and altered his appearance in other ways to keep from being apprehended by Chiang's secret police.

Zhou seemed very different from the coarse, ideology-spouting Communist officials in Yentai and down in the Flooded Area. He was warm and chatty. There was also something about his manner that connoted fairness and integrity. His given name, Enlai, meant "advent of grace," which seemed appropriate, because he spoke with such suave persuasion. On the other hand, his Communist Party nickname was *Lao Shan,* or Small Mountain, in recognition of his steadfastness. As the conversation continued into the night, I was smitten by this revolutionary leader even though for almost thirty years he had been involved in all the battles, conspiracies, lies, and murders of the Communist Party.

I was sure Zhou had urgent military business in Kaifeng, as we found out later. But it struck me as ironic that the man on whose head Chiang had placed an $80,000 price tag would appear in Kaifeng so soon after the generalissimo departed. That coincidence would have been the lead of my story. In the succeeding paragraphs I would have explained how the two men started out as cohorts at the Whampoa Military Academy, established near Guangzhou and modeled after the Soviet Red Command School founded by Leon Trotsky. Chiang had been Whampoa's commandant, Zhou its political director. Together, they had flung themselves into their mentor Sun Yat-sen's campaign to overthrow the corrupt Northern warlords and unify the country under the republic. But then, in 1927, after Zhou staged a successful insurrection in Chiang's behalf in Shanghai and set up a leftist governing body there, the generalissimo double-crossed him. That was when Chiang sicced "Big Ears" Du's Green Gang on Zhou's followers, killing most of them. Whether Chiang purposely allowed his former comrade-in-arms to escape was never determined. In any case, Zhou claimed that if it hadn't been for Norman Watts, a British shipping magnate who had fought briefly with the Communist guerrillas against the Japanese, he would have been killed. It was Watts, he said, who smuggled him aboard the freighter bound for Wuhan.

At breakfast the next morning, Zhou regaled us with more stories about those early days, ridiculing the low price Chiang had put on his head. He described the ordeal of the thirty thousand Communist men and women's epic, six-thousand-mile retreat to the safe haven of Yanan in the mountainous northwest, an exodus immortalized as the legendary Long March. The two-year trek in 1933 and 1934, he related, had taken the Red Army through the opium country in Guizhou, Sichuan, and Yunnan, where "poppy fields bloomed pastel pink," as he described them. "Everyone smoked," he confessed. "Even babies were put to sleep sucking on sugar cane covered with opium dust."

But in discussing the business at hand, Zhou was deadly serious. The UNRRA agreement with CLARA, which he quoted verbatim, clearly stated that all "relief and rehabilitation resources are to be dispensed according to the needs of the area's population, without discrimination because of race, creed, or political belief." He claimed that, contrary to orders from Washington, the relief supplies were being used as by the Nationalists as "military weapons." He then proposed that, henceforth, all UNRRA supplies for the liberated areas be turned over directly to CLARA, thus bypassing the corrupt CNRRA distribution system.

That, I knew, would be impossible. Mr. Li and K. Y. Chen, would never allow UNRRA to ship directly to the Communists. There was no use arguing the point. But I cited other problems that were keeping the relief supplies from being received by their intended recipients in the liberated areas. The Communist soldiers, as well as the Nationalists, I told him, were commandeering a number of our trucks and looting their cargoes. Zhou nodded, indicating that he was aware of the situation, and promised to send word to the Communist military commanders in Henan to leave our trucks alone. One thing he didn't tell us was that the following month he was going to issue a landmark directive to all Communist commanders to launch a massive, nationwide counteroffensive to overthrow Chiang Kai-shek. That probably was the main reason for his unexpected visit to Kaifeng.

Soon after Zhou departed, the Nationalists dropped any pretenses of safe passage for the ships destined for Yentai by slapping a blockade on all of the Shandong Peninsula ports. Even the right of UNRRA and CNRRA personnel to move freely about Henan was no longer assured. At our headquarters in Kaifeng, we could only speculate on what had precipitated this policy reversal. It came right after General Hao Peng-chu, Chiang Kai-shek's senior military man in our area, had been taken prisoner by the Communists. Possibly there was no connection, but we assumed there was because the general's capture had panicked the Nationalists and made them lash out in all directions, including ours. And the way the Communist radio crowed about his capture only made matters worse for us.

General Hao was the highest-ranking prisoner taken by the Communists up until that time. He was also their most profitable catch—a cache of three hundred gold bars having been discovered in his possession. And since this general was notorious for shooting all of his Communist prisoners, he was sent before a firing squad to die as a war criminal. Then, to further humiliate the Nationalists, a couple of embarrassing postscripts were added to the news of his execution. The Communists broadcast that it was only because of Hao's cowardly attempt to bribe his way to freedom that his gold horde had been discovered. At the last minute, they said, he tried to save his neck by offering them an additional million dollars in U.S. greenbacks, which he claimed to have stashed away in a safe deposit box in Shanghai.

Instead of dismissing the story as Red propaganda, the Nationalists in effect confirmed it by disclosing that they had opened General Hao's safety deposit box and confiscated the million dollars. But the Nationalist government's embarrassment didn't end there. The U.S. immediately protested to Chiang that Hao's gold cache had been stolen from a thirteen-ton emergency shipment flown from Fort Knox, Kentucky, to prop up China's sagging currency.

Tales of corruption like that didn't help morale in UNRRA's Kaifeng headquarters. By late August, our mission was prepared to withdraw from Henan because the Chinese government seemed to be intentionally frustrating every attempt to bring relief to the province, either by corruption or physical harassment. In fact, things had become just as bad in the other provinces, forcing LaGuardia to place a temporary embargo on all future shipments to China.

That was the abysmal state of affairs when Harlan Cleveland flew into Kaifeng in the wake of Chiang's and Zhou's visits. A young, tall, and commanding figure, he didn't hide the fact in his dealings with both the Nationalists and Communists that he was President Grover Cleveland's grandson, and a man whose own political ambitions were to be reckoned with. I was at the airport to greet him. As soon as his C-47 rolled to a stop at the end of the runway, he invited me aboard for an aerial inspection tour of the Flooded Area. For the next two hours, we flew the loop around Xuchang, Wunudian, Yanling, Fukou, Xihua, and back to Kaifeng, a trip that took our trucks at least two or three days to make.

From the air we spotted a CNRRA convoy kicking up clouds of red dust like a caravan of camels crossing the desert, only in this case it was trucks crossing the parched, silt-covered no-man's-land that the returning farmers were hoping to resuscitate with the help of UNRRA supplies, so far undelivered.

"I can't see the highway," Mr. Cleveland kept repeating as he peered down at the unmarked expanse.

"It's not a highway," I explained. "Just ruts."

"Where are the farms?" he asked.

"Most of the crops haven't been planted yet," I replied. "Everything was delayed because our fleet of CNRRA trucks that were supposed to deliver the seeds, fertilizer, and equipment in the spring didn't begin operating until July." I sensed that he already knew from reports received in Shanghai that the whole planting cycle was out of kilter. Nevertheless, he feigned surprise, acting as if he was hearing this discouraging news for the first time.

The real reason for Harlan Cleveland's visit was not prompted by his concern for the farmers in the province. He wanted to investigate the sporadic attacks on UNRRA and CNRRA personnel. I told him about the three bullets fired harmlessly, as it turned out, into my jeep. "Most likely Nationalists pretending they were Communists," I explained. The *New York Post* had reported the incident and even ran a picture (submitted, much to my surprise, by a friend in New York) of Claude Lievsay and me standing next to the riddled jeep. But, apparently, Mr. Cleveland hadn't spotted the clipping sent from UNRRA headquarters in Washington.

"Whew!" he exclaimed, emitting a low whistle. "I hate to hear about close calls like that no matter who the culprits are." But then he added, "At least your encounter didn't end in disaster. Not like the attacks made on the relocation teams dispatched to the towns along the Yellow River."

Mr. Cleveland was painfully aware of those two more serious incidents. A Canadian doctor delivering CNRRA medical supplies to one of the Communist-held towns had died of what was officially termed "exposure," though nobody said to what. Gunfire, we guessed. Soon after the doctor's death, the relocation team director's truck was blown up by retreating Communists, who mistook it for a Nationalist vehicle and rolled a couple of grenades under the rear axle.

By the time he flew back to Shanghai, Harlan Cleveland had concluded that only one of the three UNRRA projects in Henan was still viable—the mission that Claude and I and our seven hundred Chinese truck drivers and mechanics were assigned to carry out. He reasoned that since six hundred thousand families had returned from the neighboring provinces to the now-dry Flooded Area with the promise of UNRRA aid, we were obliged to deliver it.

Most of the UNRRA staff in Kaifeng, including Millie, had already been sent back to Shanghai. For safety's sake that was the right move. But Millie's departure further depleted my spirits. And so did Harlan Cleveland's decision to leave Claude and me holding the bag in Henan. It would have been different if my role there was to tell the story of a relief mission gone awry. That would have been okay. The risk of escorting more convoys through the Flooded Area no-man's-land would have been worth taking. At least my reportorial urge would have been satisfied. But my reporting was still confined to note-taking for the as-yet-unwritten "UNRRA in Bandit Land" exposé. The woman serving as my literary agent in New York City had probably now given up hope of ever getting it. "Why don't you send me more pictures?" she wrote. "They're easier to sell."

I had already sent her a macabre set of photographs of five thousand Chinese skulls lined up temple-to-temple on a hillside—an eerie image of ten thousand empty eye sockets staring into space. She seemed excited about the possibility of the pictures being published. As my accompanying captions explained, the grisly gallery, which I called "A Stadium of Skulls," had been erected by the citizens of Hengyan in Hunan Province as a memorial to their relatives, massacred by the Japanese in 1944. Buried in shallow trenches, the fleshless skeletons were exhumed right after the war. Then, the whitened skulls were arranged in tiers to simulate a grandstand of ghosts overlooking the scene of their slaughter. "That stadium of skulls is far more eloquent than any man-made memorial," the agent immediately wrote back. "I've forwarded the negatives to *Life* magazine."

That good news was accompanied by bad news from the admissions people at Columbia's School of Journalism. In a terse one-paragraph letter, they rejected me, making the prospect of my remaining in Henan for another year all the more likely—indeed a depressing thought. It reminded me that Theodore White had ended his harrowing account of the famine in Henan by admitting that the place left him "mentally sick, depressed, and filled with dire foreboding." That's exactly how I felt.

By November, the fighting in Henan had gotten worse. Our convoys were being constantly harassed, and the provincial warehouses bulged with three thousand tons of undistributed supplies. LaGuardia had lifted the embargo, and thousands of more tons were due to arrive, all of it desperately needed to avoid another killer famine. Conditions hadn't reverted to the terrible state described by White, but time was running out. Winter wheat, the main cash crop, had to be planted before the ground froze, although corn and millet, the secondary crops, didn't have to be sown until right after the wheat harvest in May. Yet the whole planting cycle was destined to collapse if the seeds and farm tools weren't distributed quickly, and there was little chance they would be.

On December 1, without another job on the horizon, I decided to make a clean break of it and quit. At the request of the UNRRA boss in Kaifeng, I agreed to accompany one more convoy down to Xihua, the Communist-held town in the heart of the Flooded Area. But that promise made me apprehensive. It was like agreeing with a friend to take one more ski run down the mountain. That's when you break a leg.

Surprisingly, the ninety-mile trip down was completed without incident. As the convoy threaded its way along Xihua's cluttered main street, a company of soldiers blocked the way. They were young and high-spirited, although shabbily dressed and armed only with old muskets. Their commanding officer backed the company into a side alley to let our convoy pass. They weren't always so obliging. Once, when the control of the city was still seesawing back and forth, Communist soldiers broke into one of our nearby truck compounds, forced the drivers to take them to Xihua, captured it, hauled the defending Nationalist troops ten miles out of town, stripped them of their arms, ammunition, and uniforms, and then returned the trucks and drivers to the CNRRA compound.

Our convoy crept cautiously around a tight corner, knocking loose a few bricks from the buildings, as so often happened. Ahead the green-tiled roof of a Buddhist temple, serving as the CNRRA warehouse, reflected the afternoon sun. A swarm of coolies quickly set about unloading the contents of the trucks into the temple, where Buddhist idols still glowered down from high golden perches. The whole scene couldn't have been more idyllic.

Unfortunately for the citizens of Xihua, our convoy had brought more clothing than food. The people needed clothing badly, but they needed food even more. Much of the cargo would therefore end up being sold by the hungry recipients to buy rice or flour. That was another distribution problem we encountered, and one that I had complained to Mr. Li about. The Communist towns were often discriminated against and handed stuff the Nationalists had too much of. As a result, flourishing black markets sprang up in a number of Communist-held towns.

Thousands of sweaters, suits, and coats hung from sales racks in Xihua's main shopping street. Some of the clothing looked brand new: Hart, Shaffner and Marx overcoats selling for the equivalent of five dollars; Macgregor sweaters for one dollar; and stylish women's jackets bearing New York City department store labels going for even less because they weren't very warm. Of course, the peasants who'd been given these items by CNRRA sold them for half of what the merchants were charging.

After the bone-rattling ride from Kaifeng, it was pretty discouraging seeing all of this supposedly free clothing being peddled by greedy merchants. Ironic, too, in a supposedly anticapitalist community. Suddenly, the total waste of seventeen months spent in China blotted out any sense of relief I was feeling on this final trip to the Flooded Area. I couldn't help but think of the tremendous effort that had gone into getting that clothing to Xihua. First, all the donated garments had to be collected at various volunteer centers around the U.S. before being baled and trucked to San Francisco for shipment to Shanghai. Unloaded onto Huangpu River lighters, the individual bales were then borne on the sweating backs of coolies to trucks that delivered them to the railway boxcars that finally carried them the last six-hundred miles to Kaifeng—provided the Lunghai line hadn't been cut.

The futility of being the last link in this tortuous supply chain leading to a black market was infuriating. During the drive down to Xihua, jouncing along across the desolate no-man's-land, I had even considered postponing my departure from Henan. I felt torn. The people of the province desperately needed most of the things our trucks were bringing to them. But then, was it worth spending another month, perhaps a year, escorting convoy after convoy through a war area only to have the cargoes end up in the hands of some petty profiteer?

Perhaps it was the combination of sun, dust, and the jarring return ride that convinced me to stick to my plan and quit. Also, news had just reached Kaifeng of yet another CNRRA scandal—a bogus bill for $190 million submitted by T. V. Soong for storing and transporting all the supplies that CNRRA had shipped to the hinterlands. It was assumed that most of the $190 million would go straight into Soong's pocket. Even so, we heard the bill couldn't be challenged because the generalissimo had just named him premier and questioning his honesty would have caused a diplomatic ruckus.

Certainly, the black marketeering of CNRRA clothing in Xihua was a mere misdemeanor compared to this latest scandal. Or, for that matter, compared to the wholesale theft of relief supplies that had been going on in Shanghai since the relief program's inception. Only in Shanghai the corruption was hard to detect. It usually emanated from polished, tea-laden conference tables, where the crooked deals were camouflaged by the most polite conversation.

On December 10, I packed up my gear and headed for Wuhan on the first leg of my journey back to Shanghai.

5

CHANCE ENCOUNTER AT THE PALACE

Few foreigners were left when I arrived in Wuhan, the former revolutionary capital. The trip from Kaifeng had taken four days—one day by truck along the top of the dike to Zhengzhou, followed by three seemingly endless days and nights sitting up on a train that made innumerable unscheduled stops. The long rail journey, however, was enlivened for me by journalist Vincent Sheean's fascinating memoir, *Personal History.* The book was required reading in my freshman English class at Dartmouth. But having gotten bogged down in the early chapters about the Moroccan Rif, where he encountered the revolutionary Sultan Sheikh Abd el-Krim, I never reached the part describing his adventures in China.

Sheean was just twenty-seven, exactly my age, when he arrived in Wuhan on assignment for the North American Newspaper Alliance. It was in this Yangtze River city in 1911 that the first battles had taken place leading to the overthrow of the Manchu Dynasty. In 1924, it became the seat of the revolutionary government. But not until July 1927, the time of Sheean's arrival, did the political ferment there reach a boiling point and then turn violent because of the sudden collapse of the early coalition between Mao Zedong and Chiang Kai-shek. Chiang then established his own Nationalist capital in Nanjing (which means Southern Capital), while his armies swept north and attacked the Communists in Wuhan.

Mao had already left. But in rapid succession, Zhou Enlai and his wife went into hiding in the home of American Bishop Logan Hubert Roots. Madame Sun Yat-sen, the petite, fiery widow of the republic's founder, whom Sheean called "China's Joan of Arc," promptly broke with her brother-in-law, the generalissimo, for "usurping the revolution," and switched allegiance to Mao. So did Foreign Minister Eugene Chen, a part black, part Chinese British subject born in Trinidad who had become one of Sun Yat-sen's revolutionaries because of his inherent hatred of what he called "the pretentious white race."

Joining the anti-Chiang, pro-Mao faction that Sheean became involved with, was a group of American fellow travelers, including Bill Prohme and his red-headed spitfire wife, Rayna; Milly Bennett; and the writer, Anna Louise Strong. As Chiang's forces approached Wuhan, all of them, including Madame Sun and Chen, fled Wuhan, taking up temporary residence in Moscow. Sheean viewed their sudden departure and end of their "desire to help create a Red China" as being frustrated "by the coalition of great Western powers which occupied the country with their armies and navies, and protected all the capital in the foreign banks."

While he was there, Sheean fell under the spell of Mikhail Markovich Borodin, Stalin's high advisor in China, who was also serving as director of Wuhan's Revolutionary Center. This tall Latvian Jew with a Stalin-style black walrus mustache, was educated at Valparaiso University in Indiana, where he called himself Mike Berg. He had been sent to China by the Kremlin in 1923 to teach the budding Communists the art of revolution. I, too, had been fascinated by accounts of Borodin's unique role. First, how he had tutored Dr. Sun Yat-sen in establishing a centralized Lenin-style organization, and then by the way he prodded both Chiang and Mao into accepting Soviet aid for the formation of a united revolutionary front. As he liked to say, his directive from the Kremlin was, "No friction, no ruction." In other words, keep the peace between the Nationalist and Communist leaders.

No individual since Sheikh Abd el-Krim had so impressed Sheean. Both the Sheikh and Borodin, he wrote, "had that special quality of being in, but above the battle." He went on to describe Borodin as "a large, calm man with the natural dignity of a lion or a panther." But in 1927 Borodin also fell out with Mao, who accused him of being a "blunderer" for opposing land redistribution. Taking flight to Moscow with the anti-Chiang faction, Borodin complained that China's revolution had "turned into a ladies' tea party."

Sheean was one of those journalists known as the "Young Falcons," who interwove their personal adventures with their reporting in the tradition of Richard Harding Davis, the daring young scribe who had covered the Spanish–American War with such color and verve for the Hearst newspapers. By using that same reporting technique, Sheean brought the whole colorful cast in Wuhan to life. But when he got caught up in the turmoil caused by the clash between Mao's and Chiang's followers, his editor cabled him, "You are sending entirely too much about politics."

As Sheean admitted in *Personal History*

I had not been sent to China to write about politics or the revolution, but to engage in some kind of personal enterprise, capers or high jinks that would carry on the tradition of romantic adventure.

After finishing Sheean's exciting memoir on the train, he instantly became my idol. Naïve as it may seem, nothing would satisfy my journalistic ambition but to become a Young Falcon. For a few nights, a recurring dream took me flying with falcon wings from one publication to another, seeking an assignment as a foreign correspondent.

The Communists had torn up the rails of the Lunghai line, the most direct route from Kaifeng to Shanghai, which is why I had embarked on what appeared to be the quickest detour—the Ping-Han line down to Wuhan, and a Yangtze River steamer the rest of the way. The fighting hadn't yet reached Wuhan, still referred to as "China's Chicago" because of its heavy industry and Midwestern location. Appearing as a miniature Shanghai, the city consisted of three old towns built around the confluence of the Han and Yangtze rivers. But its business had virtually dried up during the civil war. Still standing, though, as sentinels of American, British, and French imperialism, were the old Western-style buildings facing the wide, chocolate-colored Yangtze.

After checking into the YMCA, my Wuhan home on previous visits, I headed for Olga Kosloff's restaurant. One of the guests at the "Y" had recommended it. "Not because the food is great," he said, "but because the White Russian owner will keep you entertained."

The barren, high-ceilinged restaurant was almost empty. Sucking noises came from the rear, where two elderly Chinese gentlemen bent low over their soup, their chins almost touching the rims of their bowls. Three Russians in soiled serge uniforms were settling a bill at the only other occupied table. As they rose to leave, a white woman emerged from behind the bar and brushed past me to bid them farewell.

The four were talking near the door when I noticed what a brute of a woman she was. Her massive square shoulders, heavy chest, and stocky, pillar-like legs, gave her the husky look of a linebacker. Olga Kosloff, I presumed.

The Russians left, and she walked back toward my table. "Hullo Toots, where you from?" she boomed in a voice becoming of her size.

"Kaifeng," I answered. "But that was four days ago."

"You must be tired, Toots. Better have a bottle of UB," she said motioning to the waiter. "Only one dollar U.S."

The birdlike old waiter sauntered back to the bar and returned with a cold, dripping quart of UB beer. Olga filled my glass, and then, without even asking, filled the extra glass the waiter had brought for her. "They call me Mama," she announced, easing her chair forward to rest her mammoth bosom on the table, and then proceeded to recount her life history.

She was born in the Russian city of Tomsk, but her family fled to Haerhpin (Harbin) in Manchuria to escape the Soviet Revolution. "Three times I am rich, but lose everything," she said. "The last time with the B-29s in Wuhan."

These White Russians are survivors, I thought. Thousands had fled to China, most of them on the Trans-Siberian Railway to Vladivostok, then by ship to Manchuria. When the Japanese captured Manchuria, they moved south to cities like Qingdao (Tsingtao), Nanjing, Shanghai, and Wuhan. The White Russians, it had occurred to me many times, fared much better than the German and Austrian refugees, who also escaped to China during World War II.

Olga, unlike so many of her White Russian compatriots who still called themselves "duke" or "countess," didn't claim direct descent from the Romanovs. However, she did say that after the Bolshevik victory she fled to China with the remnants of the Czar's army under the command of a Lieutenant General Glebov. Once she started talking, there was no stopping her until we had downed another beer together and I finished dinner.

"In Qingdao," she explained, "they named me the Queen of Diamonds. I have big club called Starlight Cabaret. Mine is the biggest club because I am the biggest woman. I have thirty girls, twelve-people orchestra, beautiful garden, and tremendous business from American Navy. I wear diamond tiara on top of my head like a halo, around my wrists diamond bracelets, and on all fingers diamond rings."

Eventually, her business in Qingdao petered out and she moved to Wuhan and opened a new cabaret called the Cottage. But the Cottage burned to the ground when U.S. Air Force B-29s fire-bombed the city in 1944. "Now," she added, "when American G.I.s come to this restaurant, I ask who is B-29 pilot because I must charge him triple."

As I got up to leave, a scraggly spitz raced across the room and angrily pawed the screen door. Mama called sharply to the dog in Russian, but it kept on pawing and snarling. Wearily, she walked over and flung open the door to shoo away the rickshaw boys who were taunting the animal from out in the street.

"You see, it's terrible here," Mama said as I started to leave. "No chance in Wuhan anymore. Just a few foreigners. Very few ships come upriver any more. Only the Chinese come back."

She was right. The foreign gunboats were long gone, but so were most of the foreign freighters. Compared to Shanghai or Nanjing, Wuhan's broad boulevards were practically deserted. "Maybe the foreigners will come back," I said, trying to strike an optimistic note and beat a fast retreat to the "Y. "

"Even if many people here, what good is business with this money?" she exclaimed. "One day two thousand, the next day four thousand for one dollar U.S."

"It's not only Wuhan," she whispered. "My friends write it's the same everywhere. It's the Chinese. These people think they won the war and they won't listen anymore. Before the war they come to my place and they don't get served. Now they want everything. And the Communists say, 'Go ahead, take it.' We know Communists in Russia. Very bad people."

Boarding a Yangtze River steamer the next morning, I could still hear Olga's long lament. I found myself stuck in a small box of a stateroom with double-decker bunks. The ship, I also discovered, was going to poke along on a meandering journey to Shanghai, traveling only during daylight hours as a precaution against Communist attack. Fortunately, the manager of the "Y" had lent me his copy of *Red Star Over China*, Edgar Snow's voluminous account of the birth of Chinese communism. Snow, like Sheean, interwove his own personal adventures traveling in China with his interviews with Mao, Zhou, and the other Communist leaders.

My cabinmate in the lower bunk was a Chinese merchant of some means who, apparently, was giving up his business in Wuhan and moving to Shanghai. But he wasn't very communicative except for perfunctory *minzaos* ("good mornings") and *wan'ans* ("good evenings").

That was fine with me. I had Edgar Snow's fascinating book to keep me company. Also, needing time for a little soul-searching about my future, the long periods of silence were welcome. How to proceed in my quest to become a foreign correspondent? Most of my buddies back home were already immersed in well-paying corporate jobs, getting married and raising children, en route to what they considered fulfillment—and boredom! For me being a Young Falcon was fulfillment. But how to become one? An inspiration of some kind, I hoped, might strike during the slow ride down the river. As Buddha preached to his disciples, "Enlightenment originates within the mind, just as different things appear from the sleeve of a magician." The enforced isolation of the ship might just provide that magic.

Instead of knocking on doors, going from one New York publisher to the next, I was determined this time to take a more creative approach. I outlined several magazine articles to write that might help sell me as a foreign correspondent. I also made a list of potential markets for those articles, including: Life, the *Saturday Evening Post, Colliers, National Geographic,* and the *Nation.* The latter, to the surprise of the woman serving as my literary agent, actually seemed interested in my just-completed "UNRRA in Bandit Land" exposé. But converting one editor's enthusiasm for one article into a full-time job wouldn't be easy.

Aside from all the soul-searching, the five-day river ride was relaxing. Sliding downstream, we passed tile-roofed pagodas and fertile paddies that descended in pale green steps to the riverbank; a picture-book China that bore little resemblance to the one I'd just left behind in Henan.

Before the war, most commerce flowed into western China on the tail of the "Long Dragon," or Yangtze, aboard foreign freighters. But river traffic now was limited mainly to junks. Most magnificent were the seagoing junks from the South China coast, distinguished by their high sterns painted with decorative murals, and with big fish eyes protruding from their curled bows. During the day, they sailed along in a peaceful parade, unbothered by the armed struggle going on for control of the land. Only at night were precautions taken against Communist attacks. With their faded orange-and-purple sails lowered, the junks could be seen silhouetted against the shore in protective clusters, reminiscent of the way westward-bound pioneers circled their wagons to ward off the Indians.

A Chinese missionary aboard our steamer predicted that these junk people could never be converted to communism. "Trying to convert them to Christianity," he said, "is hard enough. They're fiercely independent and rarely go ashore. Throughout the Japanese occupation they stayed right on their boats, escaping the suffering endured by their relatives living in towns and villages." Nevertheless, communism was creeping steadily south toward the Yangtze. Several of the river towns had recently been given a taste of the Eighth Route Army's hit-and-run tactics.

Sometimes our steamer would steer a course so close to shore you could hear banging hammers, barking dogs, even the *ai-ho, ai-ho* chant of coolies unloading a sampan. Few of the shoreline villages had docks. The sampan noses were simply shoved up onto the mud banks. I asked a woman passenger who hailed from one of these villages what she would do if the Communists came to her place. "I'll stay," she said. "When the Japanese came I fled. But the Communists are Chinese." Anyway, she made it clear that fleeing once in a lifetime was enough for her.

As our steamer finally reached Woosung and turned the corner from the Yangtze into the Huangpu, I suddenly wished that tranquil voyage would never end, thus postponing the need to pursue the career in journalism I so desperately wanted, but feared might once again result in a series of rejections. Or was it that I wished the carefree life in China would never end? Those pangs of doubt were offset by the knowledge that Millie would be waiting in Shanghai to welcome me. In a way I would have liked to postpone that too. It was time for us to break up. Vincent Sheean and the other Young Falcons didn't travel the world with wives in tow. But then, what about Edgar Snow? He did. Or at least until his wife Helen started competing with him for stories in China, and they split up. All of those conflicting thoughts dissolved when I looked out and spotted Millie standing on the dock waiting for the ship to tie up.

Once back in Shanghai, I felt rested and ready for the bureaucratic ordeal of resigning from UNRRA. I checked into the Park Hotel (the manager who had evicted me was gone). It was amazing how far removed from the war Shanghai seemed. The hotel's fourteenth-floor nightclub still pulsated with dancers—mainly English-speaking Chinese playboys out on the town with their popsies. So did the Vienna Garden nightclub, where, as one writer put it, "You were likely to bump buttocks with such Hollywood celebrities as Anna May Wong and Douglas Fairbanks."

My hotel window looked out on the racecourse (thank goodness, not on the terrace crowded with quacking ducks). In pre-World War II days, exuberant bettors—Chinese and Westerners alike—packed the grandstand to wager on the shaggy Mongolian ponies, or on the better-bred Arabian horses that were occasionally shipped up from Australia. When the war ended, the grandstand served temporarily as a mortuary for the bodies of American airmen shot down by the Japanese and recovered from shallow graves in remote Chinese villages. Now the horses, bettors, and bodies were gone, and the racecourse's pancake-flat infield had been turned into a nine-hole golf course. Despite its short, par three holes, the players all used two caddies, one to carry the bag, the other to watch the ball. It occurred to me that those cute little caddies, no taller than a golf bag, could make a nice little feature story, and I made a note to myself to photograph them before leaving Shanghai.

At UNRRA headquarters, it quickly became evident that I had best keep my own eye on the ball, so as not to be sandbagged into signing up for another year. Not that the relief program would last that long, having been hit hard by so much corruption. But all the squeeze and kickbacks didn't seem to faze the British staff members, who, feigning heavy cockney accents, referred to Chiang Kai-shek as "Generalissimo Cash-my-check," and to his brother-in-law, the premier, as "Shake-me-down Soong." The Brits, however, had a long history of doing business in China, and were used to paying cumshaw. The Americans, on the other hand, were so disgusted with all the corruption that many of them had already quit and gone home. As a result, pressure was being put on everyone else to stay to prevent the whole China program from collapsing prematurely.

I could tell how desperate things were by the way I was being sweet-talked into going back to Kaifeng. No sooner had the personnel director received my resignation than he whisked me upstairs for a friendly pat on the back from Harlan Cleveland, who began by reminiscing about the aerial survey of the Flooded Area we had made together. Then, emphasizing the need for we Americans to complete the job, he pointed out that the poor farmers there still hadn't recovered from all the years of flood, famine, pestilence, and war. "Can you really quit with a clear conscience?" he asked.

You would have thought my leaving was going to undermine UNRRA's entire China effort. It was all I could do to keep from complaining once again, as I already had done during his visit to Henan, about how frustrating it was escorting one truck convoy after another through a war zone only to discover that half the cargo ended up being stolen, sold, or left sitting in some crooked warlord's warehouse. So I just sat there and listened. Finally, to end the meeting, I made my return to Kaifeng contingent upon UNRRA assigning armed guards to our convoys, which I knew was impossible.

After that unsettling session, I headed straight for the Palace Hotel bar. The Palace was one of several Shanghai watering holes boasting of having the "longest bar in the world." Its polished Philippine mahogany surface stretched about one hundred feet from the front of the hotel, facing the Huangpu River all the way back to the dark, wood-paneled lobby—the perfect place to reinforce my resolve to quit and go home.

The bar itself was for men only. Or at least that was the closely observed protocol. A cadre of White Russian prostitutes also frequented the Palace, but they sat in pairs at tiny tables by the windows facing out onto Nanjing Road, and never at the bar. However, it was to their professional advantage. They could smile through the windows at prospective male customers passing by.

Standing at the bar, I felt half elated and half in my cups. Leaving China would be a wrench. So would leaving Millie. Going home without a job was also worrisome, though one bit of good news had greeted my arrival in Shanghai—the *Nation* had offered to buy my article, but for only ten cents a word. Just enough, I calculated, to pay for dinner for two at Gallagher's, my favorite Manhattan steakhouse. Still, the prospect of an article appearing under my byline was exciting. Especially a first-hand report on how hundreds of millions of UNRRA's dollars had gone down the drain in China. Or, more precisely, into the pockets of the generalissimo's cronies.

Perhaps it was fate, or just a remarkable piece of luck, but the American standing next to me at the Palace bar on that Pearl Harbor Day in 1947 would forever change my life.

He was sipping straight vodka that the bartender poured from a tall blue bottle sheathed in ice. "Will you have one," he offered, motioning to the bottle. "I'm Bill Gray, Time–Life bureau chief in Shanghai."

Who would have guessed it? Short and bespectacled, his mien was more that of your friendly corner druggist than dashing foreign correspondent. And a far cry from how I envisioned a Young Falcon. But when he spoke, the words came crisply, accompanied by a wide smile that would have thawed the coldest interview subject.

During the course of our conversation, I discovered that *Life* just that week had published my picture story of the "Stadium of Skulls," the hillside war memorial in Hunan Province. Because the magazine's editorial office in New York City had obtained the negatives and accompanying article from the woman acting as my agent, nobody in the Shanghai bureau knew where the story came from.

After we'd cleared up that mystery and downed another vodka, Bill suggested that I stop by the Time–Life bureau the next morning, where he already had a makeready (advance) copy of the magazine. "Our office is on the Bund," he said. "Just around the corner from here."

The Time–Life bureau didn't fit my idea of the office of a powerful international newsgathering organization any more than Bill's almost mousy appearance fit my preconceived notion of a foreign correspondent. The old iron-cage elevator at No. 17 the Bund wheezed its way up to the third floor, where the smudged walls sorely needed a fresh coat of paint and the frayed furniture looked like it had been bought second-hand at an office closeout sale.

The view from the window was nice. As far as the eye could see, the Huangpu was filled with freighters, ferries, junks, sampans, and strings of ancient barges being pulled by decrepit tugs. The river traffic appeared to have doubled since my days patrolling the waterfront for CNRRA. Anchored off in the distance, the great gray ghost of the U.S. Navy cruiser *St. Paul* towered over the swarm of small craft. It was there to show the flag. To let Americans in Shanghai know that they had a floating fortress to fall back on should the civil war suddenly engulf the city.

It quickly became obvious that Bill hadn't invited me there simply to give me the copy of *Life* containing my article and pictures. He got right to the point. Could I write a "situationer," as he called it, about the fighting in Henan Province? "We haven't had a reporter there in years," he said. "Not since Teddy White covered the famine of 1943." A situationer, Bill explained, was different from a story about a specific event. It was a more like an intelligence report about a developing crisis that hadn't yet come to a head.

At the Palace bar I had told Bill about Chiang Kai-shek's unexpected visit to Kaifeng, and the sudden Communist threat to immobilize his armies in Henan. All of us there knew that Zhengzhou's capture would be a crucial victory for Mao. But somehow the word hadn't seeped down to Shanghai about the possible loss of this strategic rail hub where the east-west and north-south lines intersected. What Bill wanted me to write was an on-the-scene assessment of whether Mao might actually make good on his threat to nail the Nationalists to this so-called "Zhengzhou Cross."

"If Chiang's armies are cut off at Zhengzhou," Bill continued, "and are then bottled up on the Central Plain, that will leave Nanjing and Shanghai virtually unprotected."

I hadn't carried my own civil war scenario that far. "Don't know about Nanjing and Shanghai," I said. "But if the Communist strategy succeeds, Kaifeng won't last a week."

"Put in plenty of color," Bill advised, assuming that I had accepted the assignment. "Give me an eyewitness account that is so full of detail and color that it's irrefutable. I don't want *Time*'s editors in New York coming back at me saying, "What does that do-good relief worker up in Kaifeng know about covering a war?"

He then explained how another *Time* correspondent stationed in Nanjing had been filing glowing accounts of Chiang's military victories along the Yellow River. "Sheer fantasy," Bill added, "but that's what the proprietor wants to hear."

The "proprietor," he explained, was Henry Luce, or "Harry," as Bill called him, whose unswerving support of Generalissimo and Madame Chiang was known throughout China. *Time's* man in Nanjing, I guessed, was probably pandering to Luce, but Bill didn't go into the politics of *Time's* China coverage. "Put in plenty of color," he repeated. "But be sure you've got your facts straight," he cautioned as I stepped back into the wheezing old elevator.

Three days later, I returned to the Time–Life bureau with my report. In eight double-spaced, typewritten pages it described the sham battles being fought by the Nationalists, the stealing, the starving, the blackmarketeering, and all the other rotten stuff I'd witnessed running my trucks through the Flooded Area south of the Yellow River. I even threw in Napoleon's old maxim: "Nothing will disorganize an army more completely than pillage." It was hardly an unbiased account. But its conclusion was right. "Mao's armies are indeed going to nail the Nationalists to the Zhengzhou cross," I wrote.

I left the eight pages with the bureau secretary. The next morning, Bill called and asked me to come back. "Oh shit," I thought. "Too much mundane detail. It wasn't colorful enough."

"Precisely what I wanted," he said. "Your dire assessment of the military situation in Henan is already scheduled for the next issue of *Time*." The reason for my return summons, he explained, was to talk about the possibility of my going to work for the magazine.

"When are you flying to New York?" he asked.

"In time for Christmas," I told him.

"OK," he said. "I'll set up some interviews for you between Christmas and New Year's. That's a good time to see people," he added. "Nobody gets any work done then."

I couldn't believe this conversation was taking place. Not after being flatly rejected by the Columbia School of Journalism and racking my brain all the way down the Yangtze trying to figure out a way to get a foot in some publisher's door.

As Bill continued, I glanced out the window and gazed down at the Bund below, clogged with rickshaws, pedicabs, trolley cars, and automobiles. As usual, small boys were running beside the pedicabs, begging for a handout. I couldn't hear them, but even viewing the scene in pantomime, I knew their cry: "No mama, no papa, no chow chow." In the distance at the end of the Bund, I could see the little riverfront park upon whose wrought-iron gate, or so legend had it, there was once a sign proclaiming NO DOGS AND CHINESE ALLOWED. An exception, it was said, was made for Chinese amahs accompanying their white charges, though some Old China-hands claimed the existence of the racist sign was a myth.

Shanghai for me was no longer that foreign city filled with strange sights and sounds. I suddenly realized it was as much my home as any place in the world. And if things worked out as Bill indicated he hoped they would, I might be coming right back.

Yet, I knew Shanghai would be a different place without Millie. Most of its excitement had been a shared experience. But it could no longer be. She recognized that, and with two other UNRRA gals had already planned to spend their severance pay on an extended tour of Europe.

I think there was always an unspoken understanding between us that it would eventually end this way. I took her out to Kiangwan Airport on a drizzly December morning, the same place we had landed in Shanghai together seventeen months earlier. Goodbyes can be clumsy. "You'll soon find somebody else," I whispered lamely. And I was right. Millie married a lawyer in Nyack, New York the next year. But the sadness lodged in the pit of my stomach would come back to haunt me for much longer than that.

6

HITCHING RIDES TO THE WAR

The sudden turn of events had left my head spinning. Boarding the plane for California, I felt dazed, dumbfounded, flying on the wings of a falcon, so to speak, but unable to sort things out in a logical manner. Too many thoughts were tugging at my brain at the same time.

Was it fair bailing out of UNRRA? And at a moment when, as Harlan Cleveland said, so many people in Henan were still facing famine, pestilence, and war?

That fleeting question was easy to dismiss. After all, as callous as it sounds, I'd come to China seeking adventure and the chance to make my mark as a freelance reporter, not as a do-gooder out to save the starving Chinese. And after being rejected by the Columbia School of Journalism, the prospect of making a career leap into a correspondent's job at *Time* magazine seemed sheer fantasy. Flub that chance and another like it would probably never come along.

But what about the "proprietor," as Bill Gray called Henry Luce? Was it possible to cover China's civil war for a boss blind to the corruption and incompetence of Chiang Kai-shek's regime? An editor in chief that refused to accept the reality of an unraveling military situation? Wasn't the well-informed Henry Luce aware of General Albert Wedemeyer's White Paper? Even in Kaifeng, we had caught wind of that supposedly secret document. "The scales are now tipped in Mao's favor," the general reported to President Truman. The *Shanghai Evening Post and Mercury,* which got hold of a leaked copy, termed it "the bluntest appraisal of Chiang's declining fortunes made so far by any U.S. official."

And what about my own objectivity? After encountering all the corruption in CNRRA, could I still report fairly on China? Theodore White contended that his eyewitness accounts were unbiased, that he was simply reporting what he saw and knew to be true. Yet, *Time* refused to send him back to China and gave the assignment to Bill Gray instead after Luce read *Thunder Out of China.* According to Bill, White sent a copy of his manuscript to Luce before the book was published, believing the "proprietor" would be proud of him. A Book-of-the-Month Club main selection was not to be sneezed at. Instead, Luce felt cheated. He complained that too many of his bright young reporters, especially White and John Hersey, had "galloped to fame on the magazine's back." Of course, Luce flat out disagreed with much of the book's content, especially White's unflattering appraisal of Chiang and the Madame.

Then, there was my own bylined article, soon to be published by the *Nation.* How would Luce react to an exposé on Nationalist China in that ultraliberal publication, and written by *Time's* brand-new Shanghai correspondent? Provided, that is, I got the job. Well, it probably wasn't too late to kill the piece. The *Nation* hadn't paid for it yet.

For those and other reasons, I was suddenly feeling apprehensive about my forthcoming interviews with *Time's* editors in New York. Adding to my misgivings was a silly novel called *The Great Ones* that Bill had given me to read on the plane. "It's a hatchet job," he warned. "But it'll teach you a little about the internal politics of Time Inc."

The Great Ones was the thinly disguised story of Henry Robinson Luce and Clare Boothe Luce. The author, Ralph Ingersoll, was a former *Time* editor and supposedly a friend and protégé of Luce's. While the book's subtitle—*The Love Story of Two Very Important People*—sounded harmless enough, I found the vicious power struggle going on between the Luces pretty scary.

In the book, the character Sturges Strong, unmistakably Henry Luce, leaps straight from Yale to founding editor of *Facts,* "the knowing weekly." Stuck in Albuquerque overnight because of an airplane breakdown, he falls madly in love with another passenger, the multi-talented and recently divorced Letia Long, who bears a strong resemblance to Clare.

Thrown together by chance, the fusion of their dynamic personalities is near nuclear. As Letia explains, "He was a male who could impose his will on the world." Yet, in the novel's most dramatic chapter, "The Big Touch," Sturges is down on his knees in their bedroom, tearfully begging Letia to lend him five million dollars to keep Facts Inc. from being bankrupted by the unexpected success of its new picture magazine, *Fantasy.* Just as happened in the early days of *Life, Fantasy* couldn't raise advertising rates fast enough to keep pace with its exploding circulation, thereby shaking the financial foundations of the company.

"I'll have to touch you for a small loan, my little blonde kitten," Sturges pleads.

But the kitten turns out to be a tough cat. "Do you know what you're asking, Sturges?" she replies. "You're asking for practically every cent I have." Finally, she adds, baring her true self, "It's too much a part of me, all that money, for me to risk."

Like *Life, Fantasy* not only survived without the loan, but became so successful that its only problem was finding sufficient advertisers with mass markets profitable enough to justify the high space-rates charged by the wildly popular picture magazine.

Corny as it was, the novel made me worry that the *Time* editors scheduled to interview me might be as intimidating as the Luces were in the book.

"Avoid all needless qualms," a wise old friend once told me. And in this case, I did. "No point in allowing a vicious piece of fiction to cloud your decision."

Fortunately, my flight home encountered numerous delays, providing ample time to put aside all of my other concerns, as well. Almost from take-off, the Pacific Overseas Airline plane chartered by UNRRA to repatriate its departing personnel developed problems. To complete some engine repairs, we had to detour from Guam to Manila, where we celebrated Christmas. Then, a violent Pacific storm grounded us in Honolulu. Finally, a blizzard dumped two feet of snow on New York City, shutting down what was then Idlewild Airport.

When I finally showed up at the Time–Life Building, Manfred Gottfried, or "Gott" as everybody called the fatherly chief of correspondents, had disappeared. Nobody seemed aware of his absence except me, the person he'd been assigned to shepherd through a series of interviews. I called his office, but his secretary said he was snowed-in at home. I called his home and his wife said he was stuck at the office. So for the marital peace of this man I hoped would become my boss, I didn't pursue him.

Eleanor Welch, the assignment editor of *Life,* substituted for Gott and escorted me to all of my scheduled appointments, beginning with Max Ways, *Time's* dour foreign editor; then Content Peckham, the news magazine's tall and imposing chief researcher; followed by Wilson Hicks, the carefully groomed, smooth-talking picture editor of *Life;* and finally, Edward K. Thompson, or "EKT," as Eleanor referred to the picture magazine's abrasive assistant managing editor, whose clothes were so rumpled I assumed he'd slept in them after a late-night closing.

The interviews seemed to go pretty well. But I was left with the distinct impression that there were no openings in the Shanghai bureau on either *Time* or *Life,* even though the questions put to me concerned only China. Nobody inquired about my qualifications—where I'd gone to college, what I did in the army, or, for that matter, whether I'd resigned from UNRRA or been fired. No resumé or references were requested. They did ask if I was single. That seemed to be one of the few requirements for the job. Since nobody even suggested my filling out an employment application, I left the building glumly considering other publications to apply to.

Three days later, I was on *Life's* payroll. No mention was made of the *Time* position Bill Gray had recommended me for. Apparently, *Life's* correspondent in China was on his way home to be fired, and I was to be his replacement. But the job offer was contingent on my returning to Shanghai immediately.

"You've been away a long time," explained Gott, who by this time had reappeared in the office. "Spend a few days taking the pulse of America on your way back to Shanghai. Get a feel for this country again." Those were my only instructions. The idea of barnstorming around the U.S. visiting friends at *Life*'s expense struck me as a little crazy. But who could object? So I popped in on a couple of Dartmouth buddies in Chicago and Minneapolis, and then spent a few more days with my brother, Craig, who had just gone to work as a veterinarian in Weiser, Idaho, a rustic cattle town on the Snake River. Looking back on that trip, I'm afraid it involved more partying than pulse-taking.

Less than three weeks had elapsed since my departure from Shanghai. Yet the China I returned to in January 1948 seemed far different from the one I'd left. As a regional trucking supervisor for UNRRA, the job had sucked me into the civil war as a semi-participant, stymied often by corruption and stalled occasionally by Nationalist or Communist gunfire. Coming back as a correspondent meant, essentially, being a spectator.

There was another important difference. *Life,* my new employer, was at that time the world's greatest visual communicator. From its inaugural issue in 1936 with an aerial view of Montana's massive Fort Peck Dam on the cover and a picture inside of the first moment of a baby's life, the magazine offered both dazzling spectacles and revealing intimacies—coronations, weddings, wars, and death—such as had not been seen before. "Picture magic," is how Luce referred to *Life*'s power and influence which then far exceeded television's. Even though the magazine was already selling more than five million copies a week (circulation eventually peaked at eight million), it considered itself as much a family as a business, full of hard-driving, exciting, and sometimes difficult people. So unlike in my UNRRA days, I was now backed by an organization with an almost magical aura. It was a heady feeling appearing at some important event and saying, "I'm from *Life* magazine."

In Shanghai, I discovered my partner would be photographer Jack Birns, a burly, high-spirited Californian who was also new to the magazine. As far as *Life* was concerned, we had the whole civil war to ourselves. No other *Life* staffers were assigned to cover China.

Working for a picture magazine, however, precluded covering the war from the sidelines in Shanghai, as quite a few of the newspaper and wire service correspondents did. It meant being at the front—that is, if you could find out where the fighting was going on. My only worry was that Jack, who had brought a wife and baby to China, might not be willing to risk his neck. My days in Henan had taught me how fluid the military situation could be and how unexpectedly you could be caught in a cross fire or sniped at by Nationalist soldiers eager to blame the Communists. Jack, however, proved to be a trouper ready for action.

But where was the action? And how did you find it? Long distance phone service in China was still pretty primitive. With luck, patience, and shouting you might get through to Nanjing or Beijing. But calling any other city, particularly those under siege, was like trying to telephone Mars. Relying on the government's Central News Agency to follow the war's progress was just as unreliable. Threatened attacks were purposely unreported for fear of alarming the local populace. And the actual battles were always heralded as Nationalist victories, sometimes even after Chiang Kai-shek's soldiers had abandoned their weapons and fled. There was only one way to find out where the fighting was going on—hitching rides with General Claire Chennault's CAT planes, with the Republic of China's flag now painted on their tail, as well as the bristling tiger cub painted on their noses.

These old war-surplus C-46s and C-47s were the same planes, flown by the same soldier of fortune pilots that had ferried the spare parts to Kaifeng for our trucks. But up there I never heard much about Chennault or the genesis of his airline. As I now discovered, the maverick Texan turned out to have been a brilliant tactician in business, as well as in war.

Because of his strident advocacy of air power, he'd been forced to retire from the army in 1936. Signing on as a mercenary to fight for China against the Japanese, he formed the American Volunteer Group made up of former army, navy, and marine pilots. Their P-40s, with menacing tiger sharks painted on their snouts, proved so effective against the Japanese Zeros that after Pearl Harbor the AVG was incorporated into the Fourteenth Air Force. Chennault was then reinstated as a brigadier general and put in command.

In that role, he became a great favorite of Generalissimo and Madame Chiang Kai-shek, whose side he took in their bitter dispute with General Stilwell over the need for more American air power. The eventual financing of CAT by one of Chiang's wealthy supporters was Chennault's reward, while in what became the most highly publicized firing in World War II, Stilwell got the axe and was ordered home by President Roosevelt.

Having come to know many of Chennault's pilots on their supply runs to Kaifeng made it easy for Jack Birns and me to bum rides. But it was always a hit-and-miss proposition. The CAT planes' destinations and cargoes depended entirely on the vicissitudes of the war. On one flight, it was sixty-three Trappist monks, accompanied by eight cows, being moved to a safer locale. On another, it was two hundred orphans being flown out of harm's way.

Most of the flights, however, were routine supply shuttles delivering everything from hog bristles and goatskins to sacks of flour, wheat, and millet. The UNRRA shuttles totaling $20 million worth of food, farm supplies, and equipment were finished. But so many cities were now cut off from their surrounding farmlands, that they were forced to rely on daily airlifts. With only three civilian airlines operating in China, CAT's fifty pilots and fifteen planes were being pushed to the limit of their respective endurance and maintenance.

Flying from 150 to 200 hours a month, Chennault's World War II veterans would frequently switch on the automatic pilot, rest their cowboy boots on the dashboard, and catnap at the controls, which wasn't so reassuring if you happened to be occupying the jump seat in the cockpit right behind them. Yet even semi-comatose they seemed to cope all right with the most unusual mid-air emergencies.

Once, Robert Rousselot was jolted awake when an engine conked out at 11,000 feet. Jumping into action, he kept the plane aloft by jettisoning $48 billion ($1.5 million U.S.) worth of Chinese currency that he was hauling for the Central Bank of China. The bank ultimately recovered $12 billion. The rest of it fluttered down into the hands of Guizhou Province's unbelieving peasants.

Another unexpected emergency arose while CAT was evacuating 625 prize New Zealand sheep from a northern grazing area that had come under Communist attack. Most of the passengers were ewes. They were a well-behaved flock, bending forward on take-off like seasoned sailors leaning into a stiff wind and relaxing again when the plane leveled off. But a few rams accidentally got mixed in with the load and a pair of hotly pursued ewes charging into the cockpit almost caused the plane to crash. Nobody had warned pilot Bill Gaddie that it was mating season.

A more nerve-racking experience fell to Captain "Bus" Loane over northwest China. At 8,000 feet, he learned that a Chinese passenger was about to have a baby. He took the plane up to 11,000 feet for calm flying, and the woman delivered a healthy boy. When they reached Kaolin, or Lanchow, as it was then called, she walked off the plane unassisted.

Landings and take-offs under enemy fire were another matter. They required total concentration, particularly during the airlifting of artillery shells and hand grenades. On these ammo runs, the Chinese copilots were routinely ordered to "assume the position," which meant clasping their hands atop their heads during take-off so they couldn't throw any switches that might cause the engines to stall. But landing on the hacked-out dirt runways with the fat-bellied C-46s loaded to the ceiling with high explosives required the copilots' close cooperation. It was their responsibility to scour the surrounding hills for camouflaged Communist batteries that might start lobbing shells onto the improvised runways.

Some of the CAT flights into makeshift airports within enemy range required perseverance and ingenuity, as well as seat-of-the-pants piloting. One day, two CAT pilots, Captain Lew Burridge and First Officer John Plank, flew to Weifang, a rail center in Shandong Province. A Red Army unit suddenly appeared outside the old city wall, erected in the twelfth century to fend off Genghis Khan's marauders. The Communists shouted with bullhorns, threatening the city's annihilation if the gates weren't opened. Cut off from the old Japanese airfield where they had landed, Burridge and Plank started planning their own rescue operation, which, if several lives hadn't been at stake, would have seemed like a comic-opera sequence of events.

That night, after the Nationalist Air Force refused to bomb the Communist positions, the Reds unleashed an artillery attack that killed hundreds of Weifang's defenders, but still didn't breach the city wall. Meanwhile, with the help of a cadre of coolies, the two stranded pilots scraped out a meager four-hundred-foot landing strip for light planes on a school soccer field. However, it meant taking off between two buildings fifty feet apart and then making a quick dogleg turn before getting airborne.

The next morning, another CAT pilot, Richard Kruske, borrowed an L-5 from the Marines in Qingdao, painted out the military insignia, and flew the eighty miles to Weifang. Circling the soccer field, he saw crowds of onlookers sitting on the rooftops waiting for the show to begin. He made a spectacular, tight-turning aircraft carrier approach, touched down, and pulled up in front of the schoolyard wall. A green uniformed postal employee bicycled up and handed Kruske a sack of outbound letters, as if this was a scheduled mail run.

The guys decided Burridge should leave first. He climbed in with the mail. Kruske's sixty-five-horsepower take-off run seemed painfully slow. He did get airborne but a wing hit one of the buildings and the plane crashed. Burridge and Kruske extracted themselves from the wreckage unhurt, while the onlookers applauded. Never one to lose his sense of humor, Burridge radioed CAT headquarters in Qingdao, "Send a fourth for bridge."

Stuck in Weifang for a second night, the three stranded Americans began lengthening the runway. As they worked frantically to complete the job by dawn, they watched the sky glow red from nearby burning villages. The local Nationalist commander handed them pistols in case the Communists blasted through the city wall.

The next morning, Captain Edwin Trout flew in and broke his propeller making a bumpy landing. A CAT transport showed up overhead and parachuted in a new prop. Now, with Kruske at the controls and Burridge as passenger, they took off successfully. Once again, only two Americans remained in Weifang.

A few hours later, Captain Rousselot, of the bank note-jettisoning fame, landed another L-5 borrowed from the Marines. Close behind came Marshall Staynor flying a Piper Cub. With half the population of Weifang now watching, Staynor took Trout aboard, buzzed down the lengthened six-hundred-foot runway, and made it. Now only Plank and Rousselot remained. Rousselot, a big man, took a lightweight passenger, the Chinese traffic manager based in Weifang, aboard his L-5. Although Rousselot was considered CAT's best pilot, he piled up the plane at the end of the airstrip. Score: Two pilots stranded again, no airplane.

Staynor and his Cub tried to remedy the situation by returning a couple of hours later. The Cub set down, bounded along and—wham!—another broken propeller. After the arrival of a second parachuted replacement prop, the Cub was repaired. This time, Plank tried taking off alone, and succeeded, leaving Weifang for the first time since he and Burridge started the whole misadventure. Rousselot and Staynor were still there, but Kruske came back for Staynor. That left Rousselot alone, and in greater jeopardy than ever. During the night, CAT transports en route to Qingdao dropped flares and a few noisy explosives to intimidate the Communists so they wouldn't attack.

In the clear light of the following morning, the situation around Weifang looked better. The Communists had not yet entered the city. Staynor flew his Cub in, and Kruske brought in the L-5. The big man Rousselot got into the Cub alone. Both planes took off safely. The Weifang rescues were concluded. A few days later, the Communists captured the city.

There were many other close calls, but none with quite so many complications. Earthquake Magoon and Bob Buol, an ex-marine with two

Distinguished Flying Crosses, were following the coast of Manchuria on their return to Qingdao when they were jumped by two Soviet fighters with red stars on their tails. The Russian pilots signaled the CAT plane to follow them. "Do you really want to land at the Russian naval base in Lushun (Port Arthur)?" Buol asked.

"Hell no," replied Earthquake. "I'd rather get shot down."

One of the Russian pilots practically brushed the CAT plane with his wing tip. Buol held up his mike and pointed towards Qingdao, indicating that he had alerted CAT headquarters to what was going on. The Russians bugged off.

Later on, neither man was so lucky. Earthquake survived a crash-landing in a dried-up riverbed in Guang Xi Province only to spend a month locked up in a Chinese Communist prison where he lost fifty pounds. Buol's fate was far worse. The former marine was captured during a Communist night attack on the town of Mengtsz, near the Vietnamese border, where he had just landed. Negotiations for his release dragged on for five years before he was finally let go. But Buol died eight months later from the illnesses incurred.

Photographer Birns and I heard many of these wild yarns during our otherwise long and boring airborne hours. Some mornings we'd drop in at the CAT operations center (called the "CAT house," naturally) at Longhua Airport in Shanghai with no special destination in mind. Then, for three or four days, we'd hopscotch around to remote airstrips all over China looking for action. Sometimes we'd hear of heavy skirmishing only to come upon a peaceful, pastoral scene. Other times we'd discover the leftover desolation of a battle already finished. As a result, most of our flights turned out to be wild goose chases.

You might expect that accompanying airlifts of guns and ammunition would frequently lead to some action. That wasn't so. In the most highly fortified bastions, like Shenyang, Beijing, Tianjin, and Qingdao—the northern cities Chiang Kai-shek was determined to hang on to—the Nationalists and

Communists seemed to be perpetually maneuvering for position rather than fighting. Only on a few occasions did we come upon a real battle.

What happened to my old UNRRA headquarters town of Kaifeng was typical. Six months after I left, the "One-Eyed Dragon," General Liu Bocheng, and General Chen Yi amassed 200,000 troops in western Henan. Then, just as Mao had threatened many times before, his two armies finally overran Kaifeng and nailed the Nationalists to the "Zhengzhou Cross." But then, having demonstrated their military superiority, the Communists pulled back, leaving the two cities to stew in the realization that they could be re-captured any time Mao wanted. That, of course, was the Communist leader's strategy, letting the main population centers hang precariously on the Na-tionalist vine until they fell by their own weight, like ripe melons.

Occasionally, our aerial barnstorming paid off. By the last week of Oc-tober 1948, Chiang Kai-shek had personally taken command of the so-called Northeast Bandit Suppression headquarters in Beijing. Although he saw himself as a brilliant military tactician, that soon proved not to be the case. When we arrived in Beijing, he was desperately deploying what was left of the battered 700,000 troops he had assigned to defend Manchuria. Chiang despised the foreign press. But with Henry Luce's help, Birns and I were granted a rare appointment to photograph and interview him. Time Inc.'s editor in chief had recently escorted Madame Chiang around the U.S. on a highly lucrative aid-to-China fundraising tour, which is probably why she persuaded her husband to see us.

I had only seen the generalissimo once before, during the National As-sembly in Nanjing. Even from a distance, sitting in the visitors' gallery, I could feel his commanding presence. It was the first time in China's history that delegates from all of the far-flung provinces and border regions had come together under one roof to try to resolve their differences and adopt a new constitution, giving Chiang wide-ranging emergency powers. There were Lolo tribesmen, Turkis, and the Grand Pan Chun Lama from Tibet, a so-called "living Buddha." Ma Hung-kwei, the Moslem warlord of Ningxia, was also there, as was his hard-riding cavalryman cousin, Ma Pu-fang, governor of Qinghai.

These delegates came dressed in colorful costumes and spoke in strange tongues and dialects. Women delegates, surprisingly, were also present, including a stunning representative from Manchuria who, at the closing ceremony, was crowned Queen of the National Assembly. In all, more than 2,600 delegates showed up. Adding to the democratic spirit of the event was a group of self-proclaimed hunger strikers that confused the foreign press by gnawing on bananas and oranges while loudly protesting the proceedings. Fasting, they explained, simply meant not eating rice.

Despite the geographic rivalries represented, the generalissimo's strong leadership kept the Assembly's complicated human tapestry from unraveling. More than that, the usually autocratic Guomindang Party boss actually urged the delegates to air their grievances. And some of them hotly responded by demanding that he shoot—not just fire—Army chief of staff General Chen Cheng for letting the Nationalist forces fall into such a precarious position in Manchuria. I could hardly disagree with that idea after the way General Chen had failed to stop the bombing and strafing of CNRRA's supply ships in the Gulf of Bo Hai at the time I was sent there by Mr. Li. But Chiang minimized the importance of the Nationalist defeats in Manchuria, claiming they were due to psychological, not physical, factors. "The Communists can't win the war in sixty years," he promised the delegates.

"The generalissimo's performance," I reported to *Life,* "was most impressive." But that was six months before, and the Nationalist military situation had badly deteriorated since then. And so had Chiang's patience and presence.

Madame Chiang, it had been agreed before the interview, was to serve as our interpreter. Everyone in China, as well as people in America, were aware of the generalissimo's beautiful young wife's immense wealth, and their twenty-nine-year age difference. After all, Soong Mei-ling was the daughter of Charlie Soong, an American-educated, multimillionaire Bible salesman, and sister of the corrupt T. V. Soong, who had enriched himself at the expense of UNRRA. But, boning up on the ruling couple in preparation for the interview session, I was surprised to learn of her husband's impoverished beginnings.

The son of a destitute salt merchant, Chiang grew up without an education even in Chinese, which explained why he spoke only the local dialect of Fenghua, his birthplace in Zhejiang Province. Even so, he advanced rapidly in the army, attending military academies first in China and then Japan, where he joined the forerunner of Sun Yat-sen's Nationalist Party. When the revolution began in 1911, he came home to help Sun stave off military threats from warlords eager to restore the Manchu monarchy. But it wasn't until Sun's death in 1925 that he emerged as China's most important leader—and in the public's mind, the hero of the revolution. Finally, after breaking with the Communist faction in 1927, the political rupture that Vincent Sheean had painted so vividly, Chiang reverted to the role of a modern-day warlord. But, under the banner of the Guomindang Party, he proved himself smarter than the old-style warlords. From his capital in Nanjing, he ruled the countryside through local agents, all beholden to the landed gentry. And, backed by wealthy Shanghai bankers, he controlled the cities with the help of "Big Ears" Du, other gangsters, and secret Triad societies.

As we entered the fluorescent-lit, starkly furnished reception room where the interview was to take place, it struck me that the self-styled generalissimo (he gave himself that title) combined in his person all of the elements that affected modern China: Confucianism, Marxism, and even Christianity. Although he had become a Methodist to satisfy his wife, deep in his heart he remained a disciple of Confucius, the sage who had given China tradition, social classes, and centuries of stability.

I had been warned, however, that Chiang's encounters with Westerners were often frosty, as had proved to be the case in his meetings with General George Marshall during ill-fated attempts by the U.S. to bring Mao and Chiang together again. And from the moment the generalissimo walked in I sensed the interview and picture-taking were also going to be a bust.

A small, erect man, his head close-shaved, he was dressed, as usual, in a plain olive-green uniform devoid of decorations or insignia. But on this day at least, he appeared just as devoid of energy and emotion. The commanding presence that he had demonstrated at the National Assembly had given way to edginess and impatience. Chiang kept glancing at his wife, as if to say, "Who let these guys in?" His only message to our magazine was one he had delivered many times before: "Our fight against the Communist bandits is a continuation of the war of resistance against the Japanese." Chiang had a habit of mentioning the Reds and Japs in one breath. Even when he and Mao were supposedly arrayed together against Japan, he'd say, "The Japanese are like a terrible skin disease, but Communism is a cancer."

Either he was uncomfortable being subjected to my questions and Jack's stage directions for the pictures or he resented giving up the precious time he would have preferred to spend with his generals. "The Gimo [as *Time* called him], keeps hopping nervously around the room like a sparrow," I jotted in my notebook. "It's as if he thinks we're trying to trap him. Each time the shutter clicks he takes another hop. Asked a question, he hops again, eager, it seems, to end the whole unpleasant encounter with the two *Life* interlopers."

Not once did he wait for his wife to finish translating a question before spouting in his choppy Fenghua accent what sounded like a testy retort. Obviously, his staccato replies were being softened by the smiling Madame as she turned them into her best Wellesley English. Her facility for polishing his answers reminded me that she had been a Shanghai socialite before their marriage in 1927.

Funny things can pop into your mind during the course of an interview. Especially one that seems to be going nowhere. As Madame Chiang continued to remove the sharp edges from her husband's replies, I was suddenly reminded of how her older sister, Madame Sun Yat-sen, who as a young widow had spurned the generalissimo's proposal of marriage, had warned her, "Don't marry that bluebeard!" I remember having to look up the definition of bluebeard: "A man who marries and kills one wife after another." (Madame Chiang lived to be 105, surviving her husband by 28 years.)

There was nothing in the interview to make news. *Time,* as well as *Life,* frequently ran my interviews and eyewitness reports, and I knew Luce would be looking for this one, as it had been years since one of his correspondents had interviewed the gimo. "Harry, you're going to be disappointed," I thought. Practically all of my notes pertained to Chiang's body language rather than to what he said. "Perhaps the war is eroding his equilibrium," was the last observation jotted in my notebook. *Life* published only a brief mention of the interview. But without that last notation.

After fifteen minutes of this charade, Chiang summoned two of his top generals from an adjoining room. One was Fu Zuoyi, the heavyset, bemedaled defender of Beijing, the other Wei Lihuang, the balding, mustachioed commander of the Nationalist forces in Manchuria. Their entrance signaled the interview's abrupt end, but as Madame Chiang politely explained, "The generalissimo has asked his field commanders to brief you."

With wooden pointers and war maps, the two generals proceeded to explain Chiang's "pocket strategy" for holding on to Shenyang, or Mukden, as Manchuria's capital was then called, and how it is still better known today. The threatened coal, iron, and arms manufacturing center, they indicated, was the linchpin of the generalissimo's whole northern defense plan. But, clearly, this was the kind of rationalization Chiang was accustomed to applying to a bad situation. Nationalist military briefings rarely bore much resemblance to what was happening on the battlefield.

On a couple CAT flights to Mukden, we had already observed the pocket strategy in action, and it didn't seem to be working. We had photographed round-the-clock CAT airlifts bringing in thousands of tons of supplies for the army, but also carrying out thousands of fleeing civilians, an indication of the city's nervousness. We had watched one of Captain Felix Smith's passengers, the Mukden manager of British American Tobacco, drive up to the airport, hand the keys to his Mercedes-Benz and home to his houseboy, and say, "They're all yours."

More than 200,000 Nationalists were supposedly dug in solid around the city. Yet a few army units, we knew, had already mutinied or defected.

Some of their officers, meanwhile, had turned carpetbagger, selling truck-loads of army rations in Mukden's blackmarket. One general was rumored to have signed for a planeload of currency, then, instead of using it to pay his troops, sent the money back to his bank in Shanghai. But we never could verify that story. Despite many festering problems, Mukden, and most of its million Chinese residents, continued to grimly hang on.

Before finishing our briefing, General Fu Zuoyi launched into an account of Mukden's embattled history. Back in the sixteenth century, he explained, the city flourished as the throne of the Manchu Dynasty. However, once the Manchus moved to Beijing, greedy foreign powers began to eye the resource-rich region. He then recapped the bitter Japanese occupation: how in 1931 they created an incident by blowing up the tracks of their own railway and blaming it on the Chinese. That, he said, gave the Japanese the excuse they needed to annex Manchuria, rename it Manchukuo, and install Henry Pu Yi as puppet regent. According to General Fu, the Japanese continued to create incidents to prove the need for their presence. First, they tried to blow up the U.S consulate in Mukden. Then they staged a phony robbery at the First National City Bank. Finally, they stabbed to death an American oil executive.

That was also the Chinese history book version of Japan's occupation of Manchuria, which I was already familiar with. But I'd heard other tales about how alienated the local Manchurian population became because of Chiang's tacit recognition of Japan's sovereignty. Left to their own fate, a few daring citizens had formed a volunteer army of resistance fighters. They bravely attacked the Japanese until most of the volunteers were either killed or took to the hills. Chiang, I'd heard, had become even more hated in Manchuria after Japan surrendered. His secret police, sent to ferret out the Communists, got rich by squeezing the local bankers, merchants, and wealthy landowners. It may have been an apocryphal story, but when Mao's troops cut the rail line running south from Haerhpin, the people of Mukden were said to have breathed a sigh of relief. "Good!" they exclaimed. "We're cut off. Now those Nationalist bastards can't come back."

General Fu Zuoyi, of course, didn't so much as hint at the prevailing anti-Chiang sentiment, probably the underlying cause of the Nationalists' difficulty in combating the Communists in Manchuria. Instead, he claimed the generalissimo had always vowed that China would regain the vast industrial province as soon as Japan was defeated. But, as he hastened to add, three days after the atom bomb destroyed Hiroshima, Stalin's troops stormed into Mukden, disarmed the Japanese, and handed their weapons to the Communists. Then, Russian engineers proceeded to strip the steel mills and factories built with Chinese slave labor before carting off all the machinery to Siberia.

"That," concluded General Fu dramatically, "was the most recent rape of Mukden. Now," he warned, "Mao's soldiers are trying to rape it again. But they won't succeed."

7

OUR MAN IN MUKDEN DIGS IN

General Fu Zuoyi was wrong. Hitching a ride to Manchuria a few days later, we discovered the situation had suddenly become desperate. My most vivid memory of Mukden under siege was its eerie silence—except for the howling wind and clouds of dust that swept down from the northern plains and blinded our eyes and tore into our skin. No exploding shells shattered the silence. No searing orange tracers sliced through the ominously dark sky. No trenches scarred the surrounding farmland or interior streets. Even more surprising, no cries of starving children, the surest sound of a falling metropolis, tugged at our hearts.

"This is a ghost city," I cabled *Life's* editors in New York on October 29, 1948. "Most of the government troops are encamped near rail sidings awaiting evacuation. In the heart of the metropolis, freezing blasts whistle down the broad empty thoroughfares. Shop fronts, and even army pillboxes, at the main intersections are boarded up. Jagged walls in factory areas, built by the Japanese invaders, blasted by American bombers during World War II, and later pillaged by the Russian occupation forces, stand silhouetted against the steel-gray sky. Mukden, the capital of China's richest industrial area, looks as ragged as the half-frozen refugees picking their way through the debris on the few streets where people can still be found."

No other reporters or photographers were there, a situation hard to imagine with today's media saturation of even the smallest, most remote war. Birns and I figured we probably had no more than seven or eight hours to grab what pictures we could before the city fell.

We started up the bumpy road to Szeping, north of Mukden, only to discover that the troops of General Lin Biao, once Chiang Kai-shek's star student at Whampoa Military Academy, were coming down the other way. A few months earlier, the Nationalists had pushed these Communist forces back up this same road and recaptured Szeping in a devastating battle that cost the two sides 50,000 casualties. But since then just about everything possible had gone wrong with Chiang's defenses.

When the Reds withdrew from Szeping, they had carried with them, like a file of ants retreating to their underground habitats, all the grain stores in the region that the Nationalist troops and civilian population needed to survive the winter. "Food and weapons must come from the enemy troops and the enemy's areas," Mao had instructed Lin Biao. At the same time Chiang, who was directing the battle for Manchuria from Beijing, had decreed that his commanders had the right to demand supplies directly from the population they were supposed to protect. Without food, resistance in Mukden began to crumble.

About this same time, the Nationalist government had evacuated five thousand local university students to Beijing to save the best brains of the region from falling into Communist hands. Given only a small subsistence allowance and permitted to roam Beijing at will, they became beggars, camping out in the parks and temples. When an angry mob of these Manchurian students marched on the residence of the Beijing city council president, Nationalist soldiers opened fire with machine guns, killing fourteen of them and wounding more than a hundred. Word of this massacre reverberated through Mukden's environs, further embittering the residents there against the dispirited Nationalist army. So Birns and I weren't sure what to expect as we kept moving north of the city.

Ten miles up the road, we found the charred remains of one village after another. Abandoned U.S. Army tanks and howitzers littered the barren wheat fields from which the grain had been taken by the Communists during their temporary retreat. It was eerily quiet for a battlefront, reminding me of the ominous no-man's-land that our truck convoys traveled across in Henan. A freight train heading south chuffed by, finally breaking the silence. It was packed with fleeing soldiers. Those that couldn't squeeze inside sat shivering atop the train in their padded yellow uniforms. Another clump of yellow-clad soldiers covered the coal pile in the old steam locomotive's tender. In my notebook, I scribbled, "From a distance they made the engine and long string of boxcars look like sausage links smothered with mustard."

We decided to turn around and head back to Mukden. On our way we passed members of the highly touted Nationalist 207th Infantry Division holding close-order drill as if they were practicing for a peacetime parade. Their commanding officer had just received word that Chiang's 100,000-man special Blue Force was locked in battle below Mukden trying to open an escape corridor for them and the other Nationalist forces attempting to run the gauntlet south. "We drill to keep warm and our spirits up," the officer explained.

By the time we returned to the city, business and traffic had come to a halt. We stopped at the Tschurin Co. Ltd., the Soviet-subsidized department store. Still fully staffed, its display counters were filled with canned delicacies, chinaware, boots, furs, jewelry, and other luxuries. The Russian manager trailed us around the store, apparently worried that we might be shoplifters. He didn't seem to realize that his whole inventory might soon be confiscated by the Communist troops about to descend on his store.

We also encountered a Chinese tobacco dealer who, likewise, seemed oblivious to the dire situation at hand. He had just returned from the customs office trying to obtain an import license. "Bring in anything you want," the sole remaining customs officer told him. "We're out of business." In the huge Japanese-built arsenal, workers were furiously dismantling key pieces of machinery, planning to ship them south by rail. But there was no way to transport them even to the nearby freight yards, where all the empty boxcars had already been commandeered by fleeing Nationalist soldiers.

Most of the city's activities centered around the railway station and airports. An enormous crowd of would-be ticket buyers had wedged themselves between the train depot and a hundred-foot-high Russian victory obelisk, topped with a Soviet tank, rising from the plaza in front of the station. Some of the people were selling their belongings to raise money for a ticket, even though all of the departing passenger trains were already filled with fleeing soldiers.

At Pai Ling Field, Mukden's military airport, a succession of Chinese Air Force C-46s and C-47s were evacuating one army company after another. We were told that during this mass military exodus, General Wei Lihuang, one of the two Nationalist field commanders who had briefed us in Beijing, had managed to slip away.

At South Field, the civilian airport, CAT and the other two cargo carriers, China National Aviation Corporation, and Central Air Transport Corporation, were running a hundred shuttles a day from Tianjin, Qingdao, and Beijing. The pilots were logging sixty hours a week in a nerve-wracking schedule that had started ten months earlier to keep a meager stream of supplies flowing into Mukden, where the price of a wool blanket had shot up to two hundred and fifty dollars and a mere pound of butter cost fifteen dollars. But the huge airlift, initiated to save the besieged city was now working overtime to evacuate its survivors. The haggard, overworked pilots had to settle for catnaps and fast meals in the field-side tents and operations shacks. And as if their exhausting schedule wasn't enough to contend with, they also had to keep a sharp eye out for Soviet fighters based in Luta (Dairen) and Lushun. The MiGs would suddenly appear out of nowhere and fly wingtip to wingtip, threatening to shoot them down.

Thousands of civilians waiting their turn to board a plane swarmed over the frozen field. They huddled together at night in a bomb-blasted hangar. During the day, they stood in the wan sunlight shaking the chill from their limbs as C-46s droned monotonously in and out. For those lucky people, however, the slip of white paper that entitled them to board one of the departing cargo planes had suddenly become the most precious possession in the world. But it took more than a ticket to get aboard.

As soon as the crew of an arriving C-46 finished tossing out its cargo of rice or flour, a wild human phalanx would surge toward the plane's open hatch. Kicking, punching, and clawing, men, women, and children would then try to fight their way aboard. The pilots had to stomp their cowboy boots on the outstretched fingers of those still trying desperately to climb into finally close the hatch.

At the U.S. consulate, we found everything moving in reverse. Instead of preparing to evacuate, the fifty-six-year-old Consul General Angus Ward and his staff were busy digging in for the long winter, barricading themselves behind a year's supply of canned goods and flour. All their files and records had already been flown down to Qingdao for safekeeping. But the State Department had ordered the consular personnel to stay put.

As Birns and I passed through the courtyard inside the consular compound we encountered Major John Singlaub, head of the External Survey Department, as the forerunner of the CIA was called. He was chopping up a shortwave radio transmitter with an ax. Nailed to a tree behind him, with arrows pointing to LOS ANGELES CITY LIMITS, PARIS, and SIBERIAN SALT MINES, was a direction sign which we assumed he had facetiously placed there to remind visitors that Mukden was in the middle of nowhere. Had the major gone bonkers? I wondered. "Orders from Shanghai," he explained. "Don't want to give the Commies our intelligence equipment." Twenty-nine years later, President Jimmy Carter would dismiss Singlaub, by then a major general, from his command in South Korea for publicly criticizing the Administration's national security policy.

Consul General Ward, who had previously served in Vladivostok and come to know the Russian Communists intimately, claimed to welcome the chance to stay behind in Mukden. "An unusual opportunity," he said, "to make contact with China's Communists as well." He certainly looked and acted the part of an international go-between. Fluent in both Russian and Chinese, this large, imposing man with a white goatee could have stepped right out of a Hollywood spy thriller. But behind that façade was a tough old Foreign Service coot, perfectly cast for the role he was about to play.

Ward realized that establishing a dialogue with Mao's hardliners wouldn't be easy. Contact with them had been broken off almost two years earlier, when an exasperated General George Marshall finally had given up trying to mediate a peace agreement between Mao and Chiang. But if any American diplomat could jump-start a conversation again with the Chinese Communists, Angus Ward was the man to try.

Birns was still photographing Ward behind a mountain of canned goods when word came that Lin Biao's forward units had already reached Mukden's outskirts. "Get your asses out to the airport, or you'll be stuck with us," ordered the American diplomat rather undiplomatically.

Racing back to South Field, we found CAT had already stopped flying the refugee shuttles. Fortunately for us, Chennault had made it a rule to keep one plane on the field at all times to evacuate the airline's own ground crew. We clambered aboard.

Flying back to Qingdao, pilot Neese Hicks received orders to steer clear of Luta and Lushun. Soviet fighters apparently had buzzed a couple of the CAT shuttles earlier that day after they strayed too close to those two Chinese ports still controlled by the Russians. Instead, Hicks flew us over Yingkou so Birns could shoot aerials of the Nationalist-controlled evacuation port we thought might become Manchuria's Dunkirk.

Riding at anchor below was the Nationalist cruiser *Chongqing*, formerly the *Aurora*, when it belonged to the British Royal Navy, plus a flotilla of Chinese destroyers and LSTs. But only a few thousand Nationalist soldiers ever reached Yingkou before it fell, along with Mukden, the next day. Following Communist policy, those survivors who weren't captured were either sent home or given the chance to join Mao's forces.

Twenty-four hours later, we were back in Shanghai. The Central News Agency still hadn't announced the fall of Mukden, and with it the loss of all Manchuria. Even more surprising, none of our reporter friends at the Foreign Correspondents' Club had caught wind of the Nationalist military disaster—that a chunk of China bigger than California, Oregon, and Washington state combined had just been wrested from Chiang Kai-shek's control. More than 400,000 of his best troops had died or been captured. Yet the government was still trying to keep this Armageddon a secret.

The challenge now was to get our pictures and exclusive eyewitness account into the issue of *Life* scheduled to be put to bed that night in New York. My eyewitness report, which went by cable, posed no problem. But the dozen or so rolls of undeveloped film had to be sent by plane. And the transpacific flight on Pan–Am's propeller-powered DC-4s took forty hours, minus the thirteen hours of clock time gained by crossing the international date line.

Today's live, instantaneous satellite transmissions, which bring wars directly into living rooms everywhere in the world while the battles are still raging, make the logistical obstacles we faced hard to imagine. But back in 1948, clearing film packets through customs, sweating out weather delays, and all the mechanical breakdowns that plagued those old prop planes, provided a suspenseful climax to covering every overseas story.

Fortunately, our editors in New York refused to let the almost-impossible logistics deny us a scoop, even if it meant bearing the expense of holding the presses for twenty-four hours. They ordered a portable photo lab set up in the San Francisco airport. Processed between planes, the undried negatives were then couriered in jars of water to Chicago, where *Life's* printing plant was located. But Chicago was socked in and the plane landed in Cleveland. A charter pilot was persuaded to fly the courier to fogbound Chicago. Holding the now-dried negatives against the window of a taxi, the managing editor, who had flown out from New York, was able to select five pages of pictures on the way to the printing plant.

People looking at a copy of *Life* the next day had no idea of the extraordinary effort it took to get that story into the pages of their magazine—and probably couldn't have cared less. But knowing that millions of Americans were seeing those pictures and reading that story made Birns and me feel pretty good. The thought, too, that Generalissimo Chiang-Kai-shek could no longer hide the truth that control of a vast industrial province had just slipped from his grasp made us feel that we were helping to set the record straight on China's civil war. For the first time, I appreciated the enormous power invested in me as the representative of an international news organization.

However, the final chapter of this story was left hanging in the balance. It wasn't until fifteen months later, when Angus Ward and the members of his consular staff were finally released by the Communists, that the world learned of the humiliation and cruelty they suffered. And then only the most cryptic report was made public.

Ward disclosed that, right from the start, his attempts to establish a dialogue with the Communists had failed abysmally. He described how he and his staff were placed under house arrest, and how he was accused of "brutally assaulting" a member of the Chinese staff. Placed in solitary confinement for a month, he and four members of the consular staff were then tried and convicted in a people's court. "I, being the arch-criminal," said Ward, "was sentenced to six months' imprisonment, fined twenty dollars in damages, and placed on parole for a year. Our prison sentences were then commuted to deportation." But Ward should have added that this happened only after President Truman and Secretary of State Dean Acheson had personally appealed to both Mao and the United Nations.

At the time of Ward's release, the State Department didn't want to exacerbate the already bitter relations between the U.S. and China by giving a more detailed account of the fifteen months the consul general and his staff had spent as virtual prisoners. It wasn't until 1993, long after Ward's death, that the fascinating full story finally came out. It appeared in the State Department's *Foreign Service Journal* in the form of an interview with Eldon Erickson, a surviving member of the Mukden consular staff.

As Erickson explained, "We were standing on the roof of the consulate when the Communists came. We could see them marching down the street. The Nationalists seemed to have just evaporated, as the Communist soldiers took over the government communications building about two blocks away. Then the Communists came up to our area. I remember there was an old lady standing in the street. They shot her and marched right on by. When they spotted us looking down from the top of the consulate, they started shooting at us."

In the chaos of the Communist takeover, the newly installed government officials at first ignored the American consular staff. Ward kept everybody busy, making them move the fifty-pound sacks of flour from one room to another and up to the second floor and back down again. "It was probably good to keep us from getting bored," Erickson admitted, "but it didn't make Angus all that popular."

He also described Ward's futile attempts to meet with Communist officials. "Angus was trying to make contact," Erickson said, "but he couldn't. The Communists claimed they didn't recognize the American government, or even its existence."

Three weeks after the Communists arrived, they threw a cordon around the consulate building and Ward's residence. "To go to the office, soldiers would come to the compound and march us with pistols at our back to the consulate office," Erickson explained. "We even had to show them our lunch so they could inspect it. Then they would escort us back in the evening. Only half of us would go each day so no one was isolated."

"The consular staff pretended to be carrying on normally, though we were really just trying to show the flag," Erickson said. Their captors supplied them with Communist newspapers, but removed all the radios and remaining communication equipment so the staff couldn't get any messages in or out. "We were held totally incommunicado," explained Erickson.

After three more weeks, the Chinese employees working in the consulate were told to stop communicating with the Americans. Even so, they continued living in the servants' quarters and would periodically bring eggs and vegetables from the market. It was like an Easter egg hunt, as Erickson described it. "They would leave the eggs in the basement at night, and we would go down and find them in the morning. Still, they didn't dare talk to us."

Every day anti-American demonstrators paraded around the consulate waving signs and shouting. Erickson, who understood Chinese, remembered their little chant: "Without Communism there will be no China."

The demonstrators posed no threat, but the nights, according to Erickson, were often terrifying. Right from the first night after the Communists took control, Nationalist Air Force planes would appear as soon as it got dark and attack the city. "Wasn't that ironic?" he added. "Here we were being bombed by our own American-built planes." He then described how one night quite a few of the consulate's windows were blown out by the concussion from the exploding bombs. Two of the staff members were hit by flying glass. "I remember picking glass out of their lips with tweezers," said Erickson. "After that we opened all the windows, despite the cold, to reduce the effects of the bomb blasts."

Completely cut off from the U.S., Ward's staff had no idea if the State Department in Washington was aware of their precarious situation. But things got even worse. The Communists cut off the electricity, which left the consulate without running water. Water had to be brought in by the bucketful. By this time, the weather had turned bitter cold, the temperature sometimes dropping to forty below zero. "We couldn't take a bath," Erickson recalled. "We just put on extra layers of clothing as the Chinese did."

Each week, the Americans were permitted to submit a list of the things they needed to two Communist representatives who appeared at the consulate gate. Needles and thread were among the most important items requested, because previously the Chinese servants had done all the mending of the consular staff's clothes. It was also assumed that because of Ward's many years' service in Vladivostok, they were permitted to order vodka.

The captives were allowed to bake their own bread. As Erickson described it, "The cockroaches would line the pans as the bread was rising. So we baked it with the cockroaches in and then sliced off the crusts," where apparently the little creatures had congregated and died from the oven's heat. To kill time, the staff played bridge and pinochle by candlelight.

Periodically, the Communist political leaders would accuse the Chinese servants of taking "capitalist paths," even though the Americans were not permitted to speak to them. When one of the servants, Chi Yu-heng, resigned and demanded severance, Ward stubbornly refused to pay it because the man had quit voluntarily. That probably was a mistake despite the fact that Chi, who had always been very friendly to the Americans, had obviously been instructed to create an incident. Nevertheless, Chi continued to live in the servants' quarters for two weeks before Ward finally escorted him off the premises.

The resulting charges against Ward were almost humorous. As Erickson described it in his interview, the local newspapers reported that Chi had been treated so roughly he lost control of his bladder. Pant-wetting seemed to be all the evidence needed as proof of a merciless beating. "The entire population of Mukden is demanding punishment for the savage and brutal act perpetrated by this American imperialist," railed the Communist radio.

One night shortly after Chi's departure, the rest of the servants were mysteriously taken away. "We were never even able to say good-bye," Erickson said. "And we had no idea what happened to them."

A year after the Communists sealed off the consulate, Ward and the four senior members of his staff were also taken from the compound and slammed in jail, where for four weeks they were kept in filthy, freezing, solitary cells. As they were being forcibly led away from the consulate, Ward ordered Erickson, who took shorthand, to come along and bring his notebook to record what was happening. "I went out the door towards the weapons carrier that Ward and the others were already in," said Erickson, "but the Communists kept shouting, 'You can't go! You can't go!' Finally, they pointed their bayonets at me and pushed me back into the consulate."

Two months after Mao proclaimed the creation of the People's Republic on October 1, 1949, officially ending the civil war, Ward and four members of his staff were tried on charges of espionage. And, according to Erickson, not just for the beating of Chi, as Ward had claimed after his release. "The authorities had the findings in hand before the trial even started, so it went very fast," Erickson reported. But he differed with the consul general's account of the sentences meted out. The two economic and administrative officers were sentenced to three years in prison, he said, while Ward and the two political officers were given five years. But all of the sentences were commuted to immediate deportation and banishment forever from the People's Republic.

It was a bitter-cold morning when the Communists came to expel the Americans. "We were loaded into a military personnel carrier," Erickson reported. "Soldiers covered us with rifles and pistols, as if we might have wanted to escape and remain in Mukden. Police also encircled the railroad station, where we were herded into six stalls in a boxcar used to transport horses."

Unbeknownst to Ward during the time he and his staff were being held, was the fate of his two consular officers stationed in Lushun, some two hundred miles south of Mukden. Consul Paul Paddock and Vice Consul Culver Gleysteen had arrived there in June 1948. The Russians, who still occupied the Manchurian port, immediately sealed off the two U.S. diplomats, cutting off their contact with the outside world except for an occasional radio message. But the Russians also did their best to jam their radio.

On one occasion, Gleysteen was arrested and charged with "signaling out to sea with the lights of his jeep." He was held in an ice-cold waiting room for several hours, where he did push-ups to keep warm while Paddock argued for his release. "The fact that it was not quite dark, and the jeep was pointed inland, was sufficient evidence to disprove the charge," reported Paddock. The two Lushun consular officials were finally released late in October 1949, several weeks ahead of the Mukden staff.

In a humorous footnote to Paddock's report to the State Department, he claimed, "the Chinese were forbidden to use the old term *mao-tse* (hairy ones) when referring to the Russians. They were to be called *lao-ta* (elder brothers) instead."

Ward's release came only a day after the U.S. had appealed to thirty nations, including Russia, for help in freeing him and his staff. It was assumed that Mao Zedong wasn't showing any mercy, but had probably bowed to international indignation over the harsh treatment of the American diplomats. Most important to Mao at that moment was international recognition of the newly proclaimed People's Republic of China, and its representation in the United Nations.

So ended America's abortive fifteen-month-long-attempt to make contact with China's Communists, a diplomatic endeavor that would continue without success until Chairman Mao invited Richard Nixon to confer with him in Beijing in 1972.

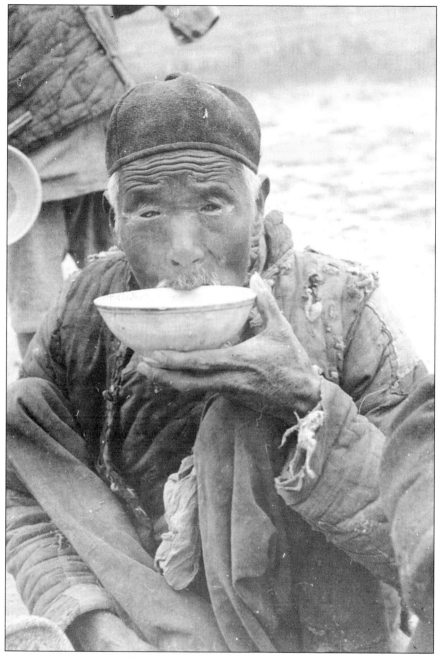

A refugee in the former Flooded Area of Henan Province eating rice soup on his long trek home to Xihua in 1947. His face and clothes were covered with the silky loess dust of the dried-up former Yellow Riverbed. AUTHOR PHOTO.

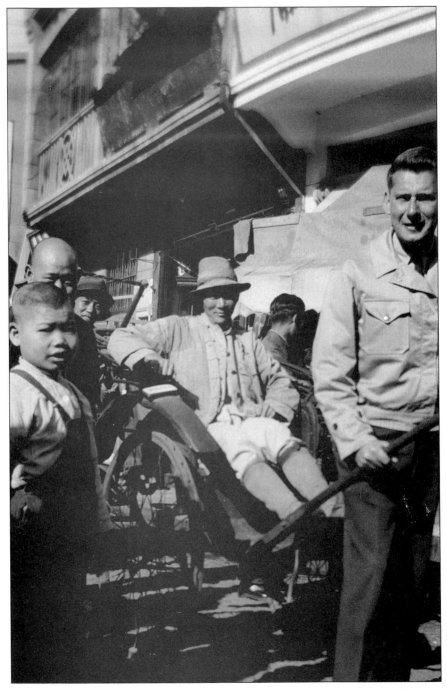

The author reversed roles with a Shanghai rickshaw operator to pose for a 1946 Christmas card. AUTHOR PHOTO.

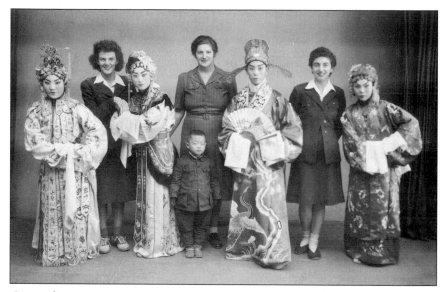

Singers from a visiting opera pose with UNRRA secretaries (from left) Millie Gokey, Lesley Excell, and Margery Soroka in Henan's capital Kaifeng. UNRRA assigned few women to this area due to the ongoing war. AUTHOR PHOTO.

The author's first photo sale to National Geographic *in 1946 showed Shanghai's 400,000-resident floating city on Suzhou Creek.* AUTHOR PHOTO.

Shanghai lighters loaded UNRRA's Wan Ching, *a former U.S. Navy LST, for its voyage to the Communist-held port of Yentai. Nationalist aircraft bombed and strafed the ship in 1947.* AUTHOR PHOTO.

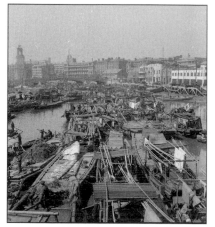

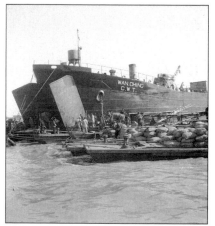

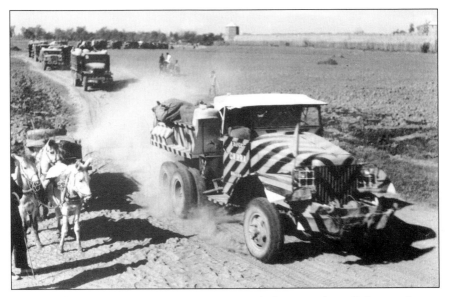

A CNRRA convoy snakes its way across the Central Plain past the walled town of Yanling in 1947. The trucks were painted with yellow and black tiger stripes, supposedly to keep the Nationalist and Communist troops from attacking them. AUTHOR PHOTO.

The oncoming traffic on the heavily-silted roads of Henan's no-man's-land was mainly mule carts, hand-pulled wheelbarrows, and peasants on foot. Communist and Nationalist soldiers routinely commandeered the CNRRA's convoy trucks, confiscated the cargoes, and abandoned the trucks when they ran out of gas. AUTHOR PHOTO.

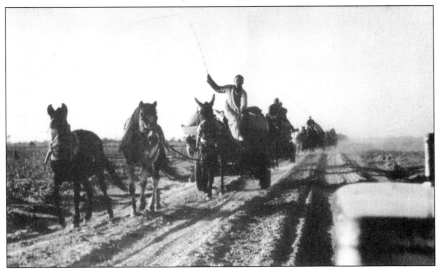

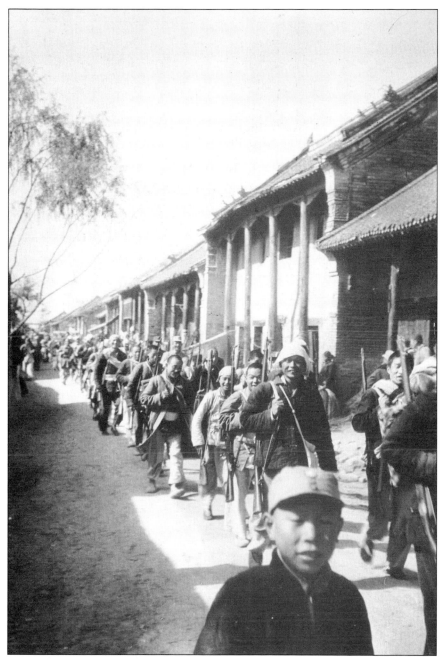

Ragtag Red Army militiamen straggled through the town of Xihua in 1947. Although ill-clad and poorly armed, they eventually managed to outmaneuver and outfight the Nationalists in Henan. AUTHOR PHOTO.

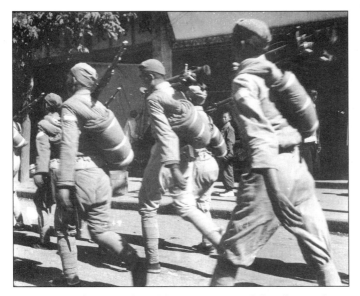

Well-equipped Nationalist soldiers put on a good show by marching in formation through Xuchang, one of CNRRA's four main distribution centers. AUTHOR PHOTO.

A Nationalist deserter at the walled town of Yanling, on his way home to Loyang, 200 miles west. A bullet had struck his neck, but didn't break the skin because the Communists had been conserving gunpowder in their cartridges. "I'm too old to be a soldier," he complained. AUTHOR PHOTO.

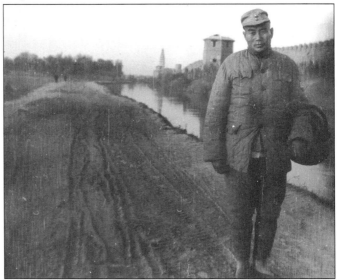

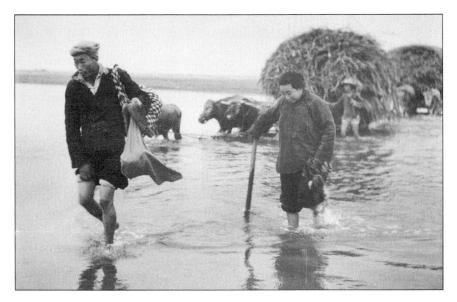

Refugees ford Henan's Flooded Area with sorghum-loaded wagons, from which they'll construct their huts. CNRRA rafted its trucks over these deepwater crossings, where they fell prey to marauding soldiers. Chiang Kai-shek originally flooded the area in 1938 to slow the Japanese invasion. AUTHOR PHOTO.

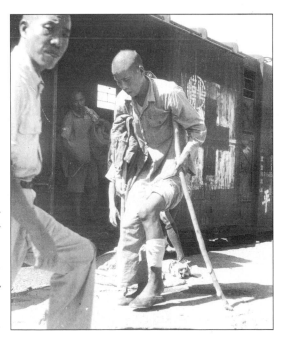

A wounded Nationalist soldier waiting at Zhengzhou railroad station for a train to Nanjing. Communist soldiers had blown up a section of track east of the city, delaying all traffic.
AUTHOR PHOTO.

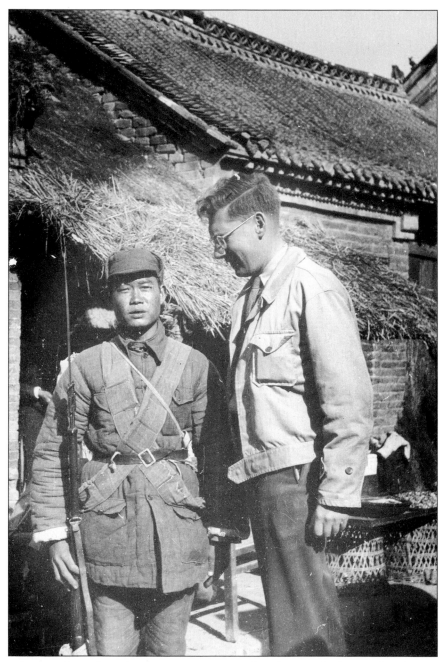

This smartly uniformed Communist sentry posted at the gate of Xihua paid no heed to the author's attempts at conversation. Either Rowan's Chinese was unintelligible, or the sentry believed the propaganda posters around town accusing UNRRA and CNRRA personnel of espionage. AUTHOR PHOTO.

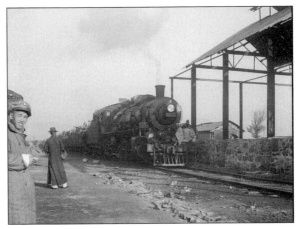

Hundreds of "yellow fish" or illegal riders on the cowcatcher and roof of a train bound for Bengbu. Those on the roof were sometimes swept to their death when the trains entered tunnels. AUTHOR PHOTO.

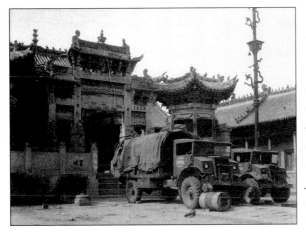

Temples were the best built and most secure buildings in the Kaifeng area, and CNRRA used the Buddhist sanctuaries to store wheat and rice before it was distributed-or sold by corrupt provincial officials. AUTHOR PHOTO.

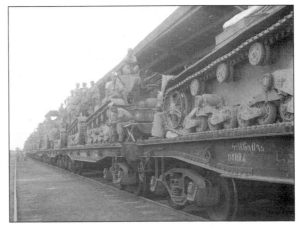

The author spent many weeks in 1946 rounding up "borrowed" UNRRA rolling stock, like these flatcars. The Nationalists often confiscated them to transport tanks to the battlefields. AUTHOR PHOTO.

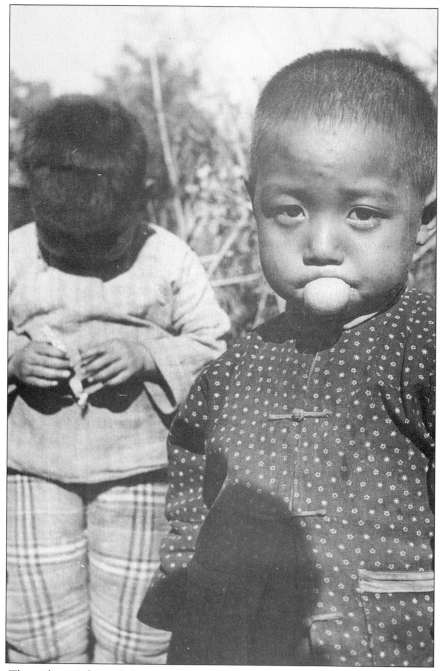

The author tried to enlighten two farmers' sons in Fukou on the mysteries of the exotic American product called bubble gum. The boy on the left is peeling off the wrapper while his buddy succeeds in blowing his first bubble. AUTHOR PHOTO.

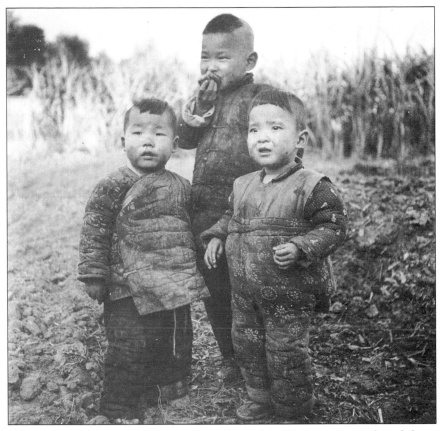

Three Fukou tots stare with amazement at the author. His interpreter explained that the tallest boy had said, "He looks funny." AUTHOR PHOTO.

In this anti-Communist propaganda poster, Yen Wang, the king of hell, beckons Mao with death's claw as a Nationalist fist knocks Mao out of China. Such posters were plastered on city walls throughout Henan in 1947. AUTHOR PHOTO.

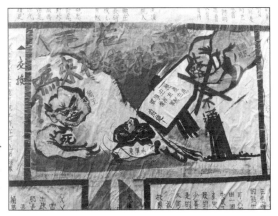

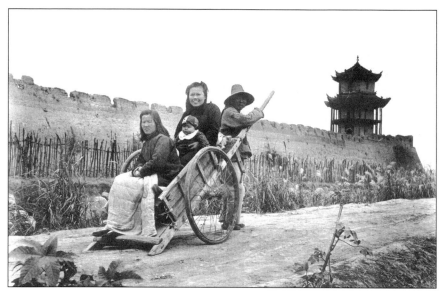

A refugee family as they circumvented Yanling on their way south to the Flooded Area.
AUTHOR PHOTO.

Hungry old women as they enjoyed a meal supplied by CNRRA in Wunudian ("Five Girls Town"). Unfortunately, mayors would sometimes sell the CNRRA food to wealthy merchants. AUTHOR PHOTO.

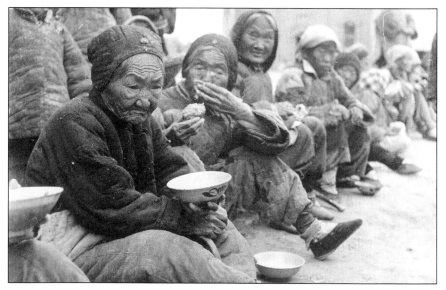

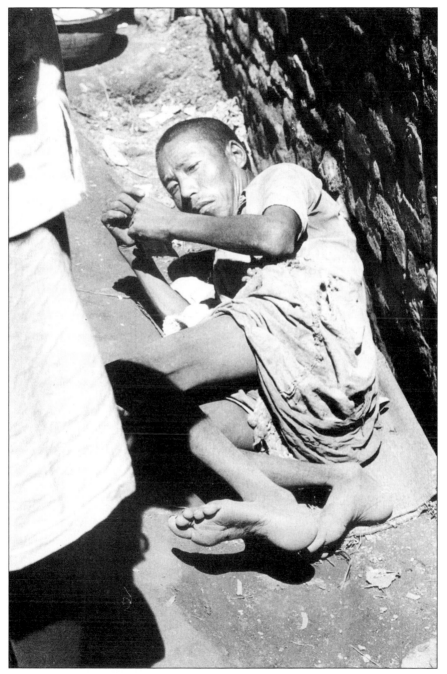

A Kaifeng beggar hoping passersby will take pity and offer food or a few yuan.
AUTHOR PHOTO.

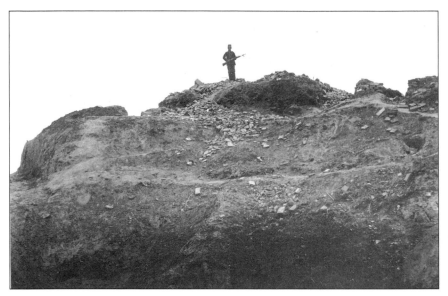

A Communist lookout atop Fukou's outer wall. Nationalist Air Force and artillery bombed the town intermittently as it changed hands almost every week. AUTHOR PHOTO.

A single file of Nationalist soldiers as they crossed the Central Plain between Fukou and Xihua. The battalion commander rode the pony. Nationalist and Communist units would often track each other across the sandy wasteland without engaging in combat. AUTHOR PHOTO.

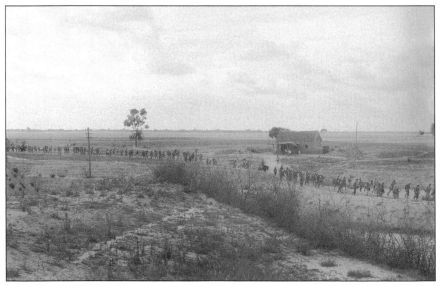

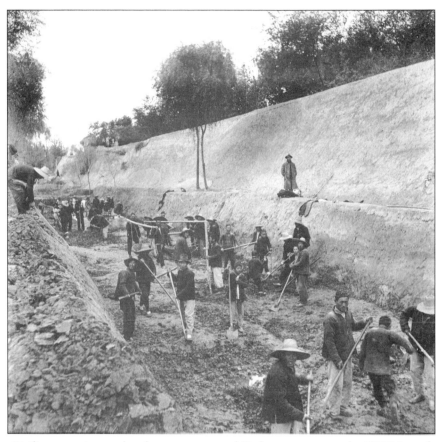

Civilian conscripts as they dug a moat around Xuchang, a town on the CNRRA truck route from Kaifeng to Xihua. Mao called this ancient market town the "Kingdom of Tobacco" because of the cigarette factories located there. AUTHOR PHOTO.

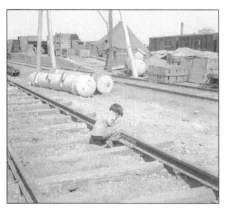

A destitute little girl scavenges for bits of coal among the ashes of Kaifeng's railyard. AUTHOR PHOTO.

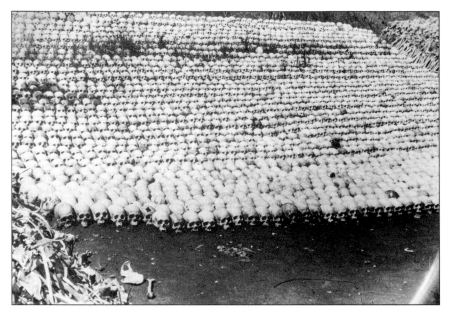

This photo of the eerie memorial to residents of Hengyang, which the author entitled "Stadium of Skulls," was his first contribution to Life *magazine, and led to his being hired as* Life's *war correspondent in China. The Japanese had massacred five thousand of the townsfolk in 1944. Survivors in Hengyang dug up the corpses in 1946 and carefully arranged them on a hillside for the memorial. In the upper right and lower left are the bones of the victims.* AUTHOR PHOTO.

The author's January 1948 press pass, issued by the Nationalist government. Before being hired by Life, *Rowan had to pass muster during a series of interviews at the magazine's New York City headquarters. "But nobody ever asked me to fill out an application," he said, "as long as I agreed to go right back to Shanghai and start covering the war."*

8

THE LAST WARLORD

It's not easy to decompress while covering a war. Our exclusive story on the fall of Mukden, and the laudatory cables it elicited from our editors in New York, made me eager for another challenge. As a young war correspondent, there was something addictive about danger that I hadn't experienced working for CNRRA. The adrenaline shooting through your veins while pursuing a perilous story produces a habit-forming high, a false sense of well-being, almost invulnerability, that propels you into taking greater and greater risks until—if you don't wake up to what's happening—you're likely to get killed.

Older correspondents might argue that they're not addicted to danger, and take risks simply because it goes with the job. But that's only part of it. Otherwise, why did some of the most senior World War II reporters, like Ernie Pyle, die taking one too many chances? After surviving the desert campaign in North Africa and the Allied landing in Normandy, Pyle pressed his luck with one last assignment, in the Pacific, where he was shot to death by a Japanese sniper on the atoll of Ie Shima during the invasion of Okinawa.

Of course, this addiction to danger doesn't only affect reporters. It struck me that Earthquake Magoon thought he could lose both engines and still land, as the old song goes, "on a wing and a prayer." I had seen soldiers in

World War II take risks that went far beyond bravery—as if they were testing their own immortality—and this is also a recurring theme in nonmilitary fiction. Hemingway celebrated the death-defying attitude of bullfighters in *The Sun Also Rises,* and of a lone fisherman in *The Old Man and the Sea.*

I was now keenly aware of my own tendency to forget caution and focus on stories, partly for their excitement. Fortunately—or unfortunately if you consider journalistic thrill-seeking foolhardy—it didn't take long for another opportunity to come along. With Mukden and all of Manchuria in Mao's hands, a crucial battle was being fought for Taiyuan. This industrial city, surrounded by some of the richest deposits of coal and iron ore in the world, was known as China's Pittsburgh. Jack Birns and I had gone there several times and, like a powerful magnet, it kept pulling us back.

Sitting strategically 250 miles southwest of Beijing, where the land rises four thousand feet above sea level to a bleak plateau between the Taihang and Wutai mountain ranges, Taiyuan held the Nationalists' largest remaining arsenal. But it was completely cut off. The craggy peaks enclosing the old walled city were honeycombed with Communist tunnels, caves, and gun emplacements. From those positions, the Reds could lob shells onto all roads leading across the yellow loess farmland into town and blanket the three airstrips with mortars.

Holed up in this redoubt behind forty-foot-thick walls, the durable old warlord Marshal Yan Xishan vowed never to surrender. His tenacity was understandable. Shanxi Province, of which Taiyuan was the capital, had been his personal fiefdom for thirty-one years. At the same time, he was recognized as China's most progressive governor, having built two rail lines (using narrow guage tracks so the Japanese trains couldn't run on them), modern roads and bridges, and miles of irrigation ditches. He encouraged reforestation, promoted literacy and public health, and published a manual for citizenship that Shanxi's ten million people were ordered to memorize. He also reformed the school system, launched campaigns against queue wearing, foot binding, and opium smoking, and even established a Heart Cleansing Institute to purify the thoughts of the local population—with himself, of course, as president. To accomplish all this, he levied high taxes. Landlords, who were hit the hardest, complained that he "taxed everything but human excrement."

Born in the Wutai district in the northern part of the province, the young Yan, like his comrade-in-arms Chiang Kai-shek, took infantry courses at the Military Cadets Academy in Tokyo. Returning to Taiyuan, he formed a model brigade, and when the spark was lit by Sun Yat-sen's revolution in 1911, he emerged as the key military figure in the province. The next year, he was appointed military governor, and, after a succession of promotions and honors, was designated Model Governor of China by the central government. But, in 1929, he unexpectedly asserted his independence by leading a revolt of the northern generals against Chiang. The rebels were soon defeated, and Yan was forced into temporary exile in Soviet-held Lushun. However, his retreat was short-lived, and he returned to Shanxi in 1931. Then, when Japan renewed its undeclared war against China in 1937, he hid out in Konanpo ("hillside of conquering all difficulties"), where he maintained a delicate buffer position between the Nationalists, Communists, and Japanese in an attempt to play each against the others.

Most of the warlords had risen through the ranks of the Beiyang (northern China) army, established under the Qing emperors. Some served in provincial armies and became military governors. Others were simply local thugs who financed their armies with taxes collected at gunpoint or by growing opium. A few were even loyal to the republic, hoping that eventually their territory would be turned into a valid constitutional state. As Pearl Buck, attempting to define the role of these regional strongmen, wrote:

The warlord sees himself as great—and great in the traditional manner of heroes of ancient fiction and history. He is in fact an actor by nature as Napoleon was.

Yan Xishan certainly fit that description, though that was not how he saw himself. Never at a loss for words, he once proudly proclaimed that, unlike all the other warlords, he had concocted a virtually perfect ideology with which to rule Shanxi—one that incorporated the best features of "Confucianism with militarism, nationalism, anarchism, democracy, capitalism, communism, individualism, imperialism, paternalism, and utopianism." He called his political party, based on those precepts, the Democratic Revolutionary Comrades Association.

Prior to Yan's reign, Shanxi had been considered one of China's most primitive areas governed by cruel, ruthless leaders, perhaps because of its mountainous isolation from the more civilized regions. One of the worst atrocities of the Boxer Rebellion occurred there in 1900, when Yuxian, the Manchu governor, summoned all of the province's foreign missionaries and their families to Taiyuan, promising to protect them. But when they arrived, he had the 137 men, women, and children beheaded. Historically, the province was considered so uncivilized, it was said that Confucius, who once traveled to a point near Taiyuan, quickly turned around because of his disgust with the ignorance and backwardness of the people. Yet, Marshal Yan believed he and the Chinese sage had a lot in common. "If we had not lived twenty-four centuries apart," he once claimed, "Confucius would have welcomed me and my ideas with open arms."

Foreign visitors were duly impressed, reporting that Yan's reforms were paying off and that his popularity with the people was real. General Stilwell wrote in the *Infantry Journal* that Yan "had the wit to see that he could draw more strength and wealth from the province by improving its conditions than by squeezing it dry."

Travelers to Taiyuan also marveled at the marshal's genteel hospitality. "Many foreign visitors came to see and were entertained by the 'Model *Tuchon*,' " wrote Barbara Tuchman in her book, *Stilwell and the American Experience in China.*

Flanked by his Oxford-educated Chinese secretary, he presided at a table set with damask tablecloths, sterling silver, garnet-colored wine glasses, and napkins intricately folded in the shape of roses, birds, and pagodas.

After dinner, guests were escorted through moonlit gardens by serving-men carrying lanterns of painted gauze suspended from tall poles. Governor Yan told them he hoped to make Shanxi a 'leavening agent' for his country, but added realistically that 'China is a very big loaf.'

Vincent Sheean also described his joyous arrival in Taiyuan after a nine-day journey on foot and by mule cart.

The old city seemed restful and charming,' he wrote in Personal History. *'The French railway hotel could not have delighted me more if it had been run by Cesar Ritz himself, while Yan Xishan, the model governor of the province, received me with the gentle courtesy of an educated Chinese.*

Not all of the visitors were so lavish in their praise. China scholar A. Doak Barnett (who, incidentally, first became interested in Mao's revolution while we were both working for UNRRA in Kaifeng) spent several months living in Taiyuan. In his book *China on the Eve of Communist Takeover,* he characterized Yan Xishan as a ruthless despot, the governor of a police state, and a warlord too powerful for President Chiang Kai-shek to control. As proof, Barnett cited a whole series of cruelties that the citizens of Shanxi were subjected to. When a group of peasants revolted, Barnett claimed, their leaders were chained together through holes punched in their collarbones. And when the disciples of a bizarre religious sect bragged that they were impervious to bullets, Yan proved otherwise by having a few of them shot. As governor, he also held family heads responsible for relatives' crimes, and landlords liable for tenants' misdeeds. Even late-sleepers, according to Barnett, were caught and punished by Yan's Early Morning Rising Society.

Despite his mixed reviews, Yan, for a while, attracted worldwide attention as his feudal nation's most likely savior. "Has China found a Moses?" queried the *Nation*. "Will he lead his people out of the wilderness?" But that possibility was quashed by the rise of Mao and the civil war, which had Yan Xishan cornered in Taiyuan like a caged lion.

When photographer Birns and I arrived for what turned out to be our last visit, all that Marshal Yan retained of his old domain was its walled capital and a small outlying area guarded by thousands of artillery pieces and machine guns mounted in hundreds of antique stone sentry boxes still bearing their colorful Qing names, such as Old Tiger, Plum Blossom, and Autumn Wind. "Seen through their gun slits, the surrounding countryside seemed perfectly tranquil," wrote CAT captain Felix Smith in his memoir, *China Pilot.* "But my head," he admitted, "told me that Taiyuan would soon go the way of Mukden."

My own head told me the same thing since a land link had been established, enabling the victorious Communist troops in Manchuria to pour south into Shandong and Shanxi. The attackers were led by Peng Dehuai, forty-seven-year-old commander of the First Field Army, who later would lead China's "volunteers" in the Korean War. General Nie Rongzhen's local People's Liberation Army forces also joined the offensive. But Mao himself was directing the battle for Shanxi from the small village of Zaolingou, south of the Great Wall.

Marshal Yan still had 90,000 troops under his command, including 400 vagabond Japanese soldiers left over from World War II. Although his men were outnumbered, he refused to let central government troops enter his province, claiming to still have a big advantage over the Communists in firepower. He could manufacture all the machine guns he needed, as well as quite a few 75mm cannons, which were delivered directly from the factory to the front. But ammunition and food were running dangerously low. Tons of flour and rice had to be flown to Taiyuan every day to keep the city alive. In fact, food was so scarce that when a man dropped dead in the street, two women, I was told, claimed him as their husband. They both wanted his body to eat.

The Taiyuan airlift was daunting, much more dangerous, because of the mountainous terrain and enemy mortars, than the famous Berlin Airlift, operating at the same time. But the press paid more attention to the Cold War in Europe than it did to the civil war in China. Nevertheless, thirty planes a day, delivering two hundred tons of supplies at a cost of $300,000, comprised the aerial parade arriving in Taiyuan, where it took some fancy flying to get the cargoes onto the ground.

The pilots for CNAC were ordered to take the safest possible approach, as if there was one. They would spiral down to two hundred feet before signaling the Chinese cargo kickers to toss out the sacks of rice and flour. If their aim was good, the sacks landed in a puff of dust right on the money, in the DZ (drop zone) inside the high-walled warehouse compound. If their aim was not so good, the sacks smacked down in a cabbage patch or on a building, leaving a gaping hole in the roof. Double-sacking kept the rice or flour from exploding over a wide area. It was a simple but ingenious system. If the inner bag burst open, the loose outer bag would catch all the contents. The ammo crates, however, had to be gently parachuted down to keep them from splintering. But in a stiff wind the boxes of shells would sometimes drift over into the Communists' welcoming arms.

CAT's seat-of-the-pants pilots followed a more daring procedure involving quick landings and take-offs. It wasn't that their pilots had more guts. After all, during World War II CNAC pioneered the famous Hump flights over the Himalayas, landed seaplanes on the Yangtze River at night behind enemy lines, and once, remarkably, rescued a downed plane in Burma by having a rescue crew hack its way through the jungle with a new wing, bolting it on, and then flying the repaired aircraft back to India. But CNAC was partially owned by Pan American, a U.S. company reluctant to see its profits go up in smoke in Taiyuan. General Chennault, on the other hand, being a close friend of Marshal Yan, was willing to take more chances with his planes and pilots to keep the city from falling.

After dropping half their loads from the air, the CAT pilots would usually try to bring their lightened C-46s in for a hot landing. The trick was to zoom in fast, jam on the brakes, dump the cargo out onto the runway, and then take off again before Communist mortars bracketed the plane. The CAT planes rarely got away without an enemy shell or two kicking up a cloud of dust close by on the airstrip and without the marshal's artillery responding. At dawn and dusk, the muzzle blast of his big guns could be seen flashing all around the field. When the Communist mortar shells finally pitted the runway so badly it couldn't be used, Yan's soldiers, assisted by civilian work crews, scraped out a new strip closer to the city.

Birns and I, having flown to Taiyuan several times before, knew the landing routine. The plane's approach was usually made at about 10,000 feet, out of range of the Communist artillery ringing the city. But it would change headings and altitudes several times—a procedure called "waltzing" by RAF pilots during World War II used to confuse German antiaircraft gunners. From that high we could look down and see the puffs from Communist mortars bursting just short of the city wall. We could also see the armies of coolies, small as ants, digging moats and new gun emplacements, as if those reinforced defenses could stave off Mao Zedong's 80,000 attackers. From inside the city wall, the tall stacks of the steel smelters belched sickly yellow clouds, inadvertently laying down a protective smokescreen over the airstrip.

The footrace to and from the airstrip was the hairiest part of every visit. Running and ducking through the forest of pillboxes and rabbit warren of trenches, we were spurred on by the ear-splitting explosions of mortars and machine guns. No matter how far away a shell exploded, it would send us sprawling into the nearest ditch. But on each trip we would stay in Taiyuan only four or five hours photographing the city's defenses as fast as we could, but always making certain there was at least one more CAT plane coming back before nightfall on which we could hitch a return ride to Tianjin or Qingdao.

In the comparative calm behind the city's high walls, we had already photographed just about everything of interest in Yan's military-industrial complex: the steel mill, the locomotive factory, the arsenal, the machine-tool factory, and the improvised hospital set up in the former middle school, where more than one thousand crudely bandaged soldiers hobbled in and out. The great number of wounded—not seen in Mukden, where Chiang's soldiers surrendered without a fight—was proof of Marshal Yan's determination to defend his fiefdom. However, we had never been allowed to interview the man himself, or even take his picture, although he was well aware of our presence.

Perhaps the old Marshal sensed this might be our last visit and his last opportunity to voice his hatred of the Communists in *Life*. We were shooting some of the outlying pillboxes, enclosed by coils of barbed wire and manned by frightened young privates, when an aide suddenly appeared with a handwritten invitation, as if we were being summoned to one of the marshal's fancy peacetime parties.

Yan Xishan greeted us in the small, homey anteroom of his headquarters, which was furnished with overstuffed chairs and handsomely carved tables. Several cloisonné boxes containing Philip Morris cigarettes were left open for his guests. Suffering from diabetes, as well as from the Communists' gradual encroachment, the sixty-six-year-old marshal looked exhausted. Decorated with five rows of campaign ribbons, his uniform hung from a body that he complained had recently lost twenty pounds. But when he spoke of his determination to hold Taiyuan at all costs, his expression changed. His eyes suddenly lighted, and I recognized the canny warlord who had foiled the Communists right after World War II by dashing back into Taiyuan in an armored car under Japanese protection and seizing the strategic rail lines that radiate from the city.

Yan then proceeded to outline Taiyuan's strategic position. He explained how his province was rich in natural resources, yet remote enough to guarantee immunity from incursions by other warlords. Fortunately, he said, Shanxi also had no "fatal rivers" deep enough for foreign gunboats to steam up on from the sea. Nevertheless, he claimed to know how to capitalize on Western skills, having welcomed French, German, and Swedish engineers ("less dangerous than British, Russians, and Japanese") to assist him in building roads, drilling artesian wells, and lighting the streets. And, with introductions arranged by H. H. Kung, Chiang Kai-shek's wealthy brother-in-law and a Shanxi native, Yan said he had been able to attract important foreign investors, including the Standard Oil Company.

Always the shrewd player, the wily old Marshal also told Birns and me how in the early days of the war against the Communists he had been prepared to defend more than just Taiyuan. He'd concocted a desperate recipe, he explained, for helping Chiang Kai-shek save China. Its two main ingredients were, first, a mercenary army of Japanese foot soldiers to augment the thousands of able-bodied men and women conscripts in his so-called Soldier-Farmer Unification Program, who, if nothing else, were trained to use a rifle; and second, a volunteer American air force patterned after the Flying Tigers and commanded by his old friend General Claire Chennault. "The trouble with the Nationalist B-25s," Yan complained, "is they bomb and strafe from too high." I was suddenly reminded of the high-flying Italian planes that came every night and bombed the *John Harvard* and other cargo ships anchored in Algiers harbor. The Italians never flew lower than 10,000 feet, and, according to Yan, neither did the Nationalist air force pilots.

"One low-flying U.S. plane with napalm," the marshal added, "could clean out all the Communists around here in three days." He didn't seem to take into account that the Red armies in their caves and tunnels were well protected from air attacks. But we didn't refute his wildly impractical plan, as it would have interrupted his running commentary and Jack's picture-taking.

Besides, Yan realized it would take U.S. funds to pay for all those volunteers, and he knew that was contrary to American policy. Yet he said he wanted our magazine's readers to understand that, given the right kind of military personnel, he was sure Chiang Kai-shek's forces could keep on fighting.

The old marshal next led us into his private office. On his desk was a cardboard shoebox filled with five hundred white potassium cyanide capsules. "See these?" he said, pointing at the pills. "They're for my five hundred commanders to swallow if the Communist bandits capture Taiyuan." Before closing the box, he pointed to a single black capsule amid all the white ones. "That one's for me," he explained.

Coming from a warlord known to have collaborated extensively with the Japanese, this vow sounded hollow indeed. But Marshal Yan swore he would kill himself rather than surrender. Not only would he keep the Communists from taking him alive, he said, he would not even let them find his body. He opened a closet containing several cans of gasoline. "After I swallow the poison," he explained, "I will set fire to this room."

Getting back to the airstrip proved even hairier than our wild dash into town. Earlier that evening, Communist forces had penetrated within two miles of the field and were lobbing mortar shells at the lone CAT plane left there with its propellers turning and ready for take-off, although it still wasn't completely unloaded. The first mortar exploded about a thousand yards away. The second shell kicked up a brown cloud of dust on the dirt runway two hundred feet behind the plane. Seconds later, a third shell burst about a hundred and fifty feet in front of the fat-bellied C-46, which the Communists obviously now considered a sitting duck ready to be destroyed.

"They've got us bracketed," yelled Captain Bill Gaddie as Birns and I dove headfirst into the open hatch. With the hatch still open and half the cargo still aboard, Gaddie gunned the plane down the runway.

As the lumbering C-46 gained altitude, we saw a shell explode on the center of the runway directly beneath us. Not all of the take-offs that day had been so clean. After landing back in Qingdao, we were told that a CAT plane returning an hour earlier was found to have fifty shrapnel holes in its fuselage. On another take off several days later, Earthquake Magoon lost an engine, but made it back to the airstrip unscathed amid a shower of orange tracers. A CNAC pilot was even luckier. He was shot down, but managed to crash-land on a farm plot inside the Taiyuan perimeter.

As we headed northeast for Qingdao, I looked down on the spiderweb of trenches and bunkers radiating out from the walled city and wondered if the potassium cyanide worked fast enough so that Yan would already be dead before the gasoline flames consumed his body. But, as might be expected, he never did put the black pill to a test.

In April 1949, at the moment the Communists were launching their final and fatal ground attack on Taiyuan, Yan Xishan appeared unexpectedly in Nanjing to plead with the central government for more food and ammunition. "Fly me home," he begged pilot Lew Burridge, who had become CAT's regional operations chief.

"Impossible," Burridge explained. "The Communists have captured the airstrip."

"Then I'll parachute in," insisted the old marshal.

"I'm sure he was serious," claimed Burridge. "But I wasn't going to let him commit suicide. Not that way. The Commies would have blasted him out of the sky."

In any case, he would have been too late. General Peng Dehai's troops had already breached Taiyuan's forty-foot-thick wall and poured into the city, fighting hand-to-hand in the streets on their way to occupying Yan's headquarters. The marshal's son-in-law and the police chief were last seen trudging down the street together, tied to a rope.

But Marshal Yan Xishan's civil war role had not ended. He was ordered to Guangzhou (Canton), where he briefly served as premier of what was left of Nationalist China, before finally joining Chiang Kai-shek in Taiwan. He died there of a heart attack in 1960 without the bitter taste of potassium cyanide in his mouth. More than four hundred of Yan's lieutenants, including his nephew, had manfully swallowed their poison capsules.

9

A TURNCOAT SAVES BEIJING

With Mukden lost and Taiyuan still hanging by the thread of its precarious airlift, Jack Birns and I turned our attention to Beijing. We hoped to capitalize on the connection we'd established with General Fu Zuoyi following our interview with the generalissimo. At that time, Fu had promised to escort us on a tour of Beijing's defenses. And I had promised *Life* to write a profile of this key military figure, on whom the fate of the historic city depended.

When we tried to take the bluff fifty-two-year-old general up on his offer, he was either too pressed or couldn't be bothered because Chiang was no longer present to prod him. A couple of recent setbacks, we surmised, had contributed to his reluctance to see us. First of all, his crack divisions, coming from Inner Mongolia, had been nailed down by the Communists. That forced him to rely on poorly trained local units to defend Beijing—a double-barreled problem that reminded me of the old Chinese proverb, "Good iron is not used for nails, or good men for soldiers." Also, since the flow of supplies from the central government had slowed, many speculated that the generalissimo might have already ceded the northeast provinces to the Communists. Then there was the crushing disappointment of the U.S. presidential election.

Three days after Mukden fell, Harry Truman defeated the highly favored Republican candidate, Governor Thomas E. Dewey, in one of America's greatest political upsets. During the campaign, Dewey had advocated stepping up military aid to China, while Truman, the stubborn "show me" Missourian, claimed the U.S. had already squandered $2 billion in arms for the Nationalists since the end of World War II. He opposed giving China one more plane or tank. "Chiang Kai-shek's armies couldn't fight their way out of a brothel," the pithy president had been heard to remark. I remember how shocked Beijing's foreign community was when it awakened to the banner headline in the English-language *Peking Chronicle: TRUMAN RE-ELECTED* (a slight mistake, since he'd taken office upon Roosevelt's death). Only days after the election, rumors flew that Fu was secretly negotiating the city's surrender.

For almost a year, Beijing had been a Nationalist island serenely going about its business in spite of the war. Now, suddenly, its two million inhabitants were startled to learn that Lin Biao's soldiers, rearmed with American equipment captured in Mukden, were pouring south through the Shanhaiguan corridor, spreading like a bloodstain over northern China. Yet nobody could conceive of a modern army sweeping into Beijing, as Genghis Khan's Mongol legions had done centuries before. Not even the Communist Bandits, it was believed, would dare to desecrate the architectural triumphs and precious Ming Dynasty heirlooms in China's ancient capital.

"Fu Zuoyi holds a beautifully delicate and priceless vase in his fingers," is the way the people put it. "If the Communists try to take it by force, it will be smashed."

This concern for the city's fragility probably helped to spread more surrender rumors. So Birns and I decided to relax and hang around Beijing for a while to see what happened. There was still a chance that General Fu would relent and let us photograph and interview him. Besides, a little free time would give me the chance to bone up on this man holding the "priceless vase" in his fingers.

Fu, a large, shambling man, I discovered, began his military training in Shanxi Province as a protégé of Yan Xishan. Then, following his mentor's example, he turned Suiyuan province in Inner Mongolia into his own private fiefdom. Politically he was considered progressive, at least compared to the other Nationalist commanders. His reputation was further enhanced by successful hit-and-run raids against the Japanese and by an early victory over the Communists when he captured Zhangjiakou, or Kalgan, as Westerners called the camel caravan center at the edge of the Mongolian plateau. Although Fu had never been one of the generalissimo's cronies, his leadership ability so impressed Chiang that he was given command of the Northern Bandit Suppression headquarters. Fu had even won the begrudging praise of Mao Zedong. "We know we can beat him in battle," the Communist leader was reported to have said. "But we'd rather not try."

While fighting his battles, General Fu never forgot the safety and welfare of the civilian populace. Before the Communists retreated from Kalgan, they set it on fire. Fu calmly went about rebuilding the city, earning the friendship of its citizens, who were unaccustomed to sympathy from Nationalist commanders. Beijing's citizens, therefore, counted on Fu to show them the same consideration and spare their city from a prolonged and destructive fight. They knew Mao had already ordered his most trusted military commander, General Lin Biao, to cross over the Great Wall and position his troops in the Beijing-Tianjin area. But, so far, Mao had not given orders to attack. The eerie peace left Fu wondering what to expect.

He didn't know that six thousand miles away, in the Kremlin, Stalin was worried that the sudden spate of Communist victories in China might impinge on Soviet geopolitical interests. The Russian leader feared that if Mao's forces continued their onslaught, the U.S. might intervene militarily. So, shortly before the fall of Mukden, he had sent Anastas Mikoyan, a senior member of the Soviet politburo, on a secret mission to "talk with Comrade Mao" to try to persuade him not to go for a "complete victory," but rather content himself with control of north China.

Mao, however, rejected this proposal, deciding instead to isolate Tianjin and Beijing while the battle progressed for control of the south. He realized, though, that by waiting to attack, the two large northern centers could face angry rebellions from within, precipitated by underground agitators already staging rallies against the swelling unemployment and falling wages. To quell potential trouble in the streets, Mao cleverly dispatched secret agents dressed as wounded Nationalist soldiers.

Fu Zuoyi seemed confused by Mao's strategy. He still had 350,000 troops under his command, but if the Communist armies intended to bypass Beijing and apply Mao's well-known tactic of leaving it hanging on the vine, he had little to gain by breaking out of the Beijing perimeter and heading south to join Chiang's forces, which were protecting the Yangtze River valley. Fu finally decided to concentrate his forces around Beijing and Tianjin and wait. Jack Birns and I decided to do the same thing.

For us, the serene sights and sounds of Beijing came as a welcome relief from the hectic days spent covering Mukden and Taiyuan. It was reassuring to see members of the scholar class, which had risen to a state of nobility under the emperors, looking and acting so normal. In the Imperial parks, we watched professors and clerks clad in long gowns performing shadow boxing exercises, a nonbelligerent mixture of pugilism and ballet performed to relax the mind and body; large groups of spry ladies and gentlemen practicing their early morning tai chi routines around the Temple of Heaven, as wizened old men flew birds on a string as if they were kites; and children tickled caged crickets with a horse hair to make them sing. Still playing in theaters were those discordant musical dramas called "operas" that resisted the most elemental lessons of harmony. And, as always, the streets were full of food vendors, jugglers, and beggars.

To record these peaceful scenes, *Life* had flown in the acclaimed French photographer Henri Cartier-Bresson, figuring it was perhaps the last time the magazine would have access to the beauty and pageantry of the Forbidden City. Bill Churchill, our assignment editor in New York, cabled Jack and me: "Relax and be tourists for a couple of days."

We quickly got bored relaxing. So, to kill time while waiting for General Fu Zuoyi, we began photographing an unsolicited color story for the magazine on a famous old painter known to Americans living in Beijing as the "Grandpa Moses of China."

The deaf eighty-year-old artist called himself by many other strange names: "Old Man of the Apricot Orchard," "Hut on Chieh Shan Mountain," and "The Man Long Separated from the Studio of Eight Ink Stones." But to the Chinese, any of those names signed with slender brush strokes on pieces of thin bamboo paper were immediately recognized as belonging to Qi Baishi.

That, however, was not the name he told us he started with. Many years before, he was plain Chih Huang, a carpenter's apprentice from Hunan Province. Coming home from work one day, he collected some shrimp, crabs, crickets, and tiny bugs and put them in a bottle. "I observed these little animals with my eye," he said, explaining the unusual assortment of creatures populating the scrolls on the wall of his studio. "Then I put them into my heart."

One by one, he painted their portraits. And one by one, to his great surprise, he sold what he painted. "Only the rich get to see beautiful landscapes," claimed Qi. "But every rickshaw boy recognizes on sight a shrimp or a crab." Apparently, he wanted his work to be appreciated by the poor, though it was the rich who had raised the price of his paintings from $1 to $15 a square foot.

At that time, art in China was frequently priced according to its size. Today, those same paintings by Qi Baishi sell in the US for twenty to twenty-five thousand dollars each. (Qi dashed off one and gave it to me that, I'm horrified to say, I can't find.)

At first, Qi flatly refused to be photographed. "I'm very sad," he moaned. "Because of my success, the rest of my family won't go out and work." Thirty relatives, he claimed, were living with him in his rambling house, and that didn't appear to be an exaggeration. While we were there, ducks and relatives alike wandered or waddled in and out. And he complained of supporting twenty more relatives back in Hunan.

"To support everyone, I must work fast," said Qi, whose wispy white beard and high, reedy voice belied the sure, swift strokes with which he painted. The slightest error in wetting or pressing the brush would have made a smear that meant starting over. But, while we were there, he never missed.

His nimble fingers could finish a masterful scroll in less than twenty minutes. But after each one, he would hobble over to a chair to relax while his nurse took his pulse on both wrists. She also stood behind him while he painted, patiently handing him his brushes or his "chop" (a carved ivory stamp engraved with the Chinese characters of the person's name) to sign a finished scroll.

I asked Qi if he would keep on painting if the Communists captured Beijing. He didn't fear the Communists, he said. His only worry was that somebody might steal his paints. So he kept them locked up, carrying the key on a rope around his waist. "I'm too old for the Communists to convert," he said as we were leaving. "If they try, I'll take them for a drive into the country outside Beijing to a quiet place where there is already a stone on which are carved the words: "The grave of Qi Baishi.""

As we continued to wait for General Fu, it became apparent that he planned to use political weapons instead of guns to try to save Beijing. His soldiers seemed aware of that decision, and after firing a few perfunctory shots, began fading away from the city's perimeter. Some of them defected and went home. Others rapidly retreated through the massive gates as the Communists closed in around the city. Once the lines were drawn, the chance of any serious fighting no longer seemed probable.

One day, wandering out to the front, Birns and I were surprised to see farmers strolling idly through their fields gathering winter cabbages in the no-man's-land just ahead of the Communist trenches. A dire food shortage had already gripped Beijing, and the cabbages were gold even though airdrops of flour and rice had recently been initiated. One of the city's few civilian casualties during the war was a passerby killed by a falling bag of flour.

We were supposed to be covering what our editors in New York referred to as the "coming battle for Beijing." But there was no fighting, or the prospect of any, to photograph. So, still hoping to catch up with General Fu, we busied ourselves shooting another offbeat feature—this one on James Wong Howe, the famous Hollywood cameraman, who showed up unexpectedly in Beijing to film *Rickshaw Boy.*

The movie was based on the novelist Lau Shaw's 1947 bestseller. Howe, a Chinese-American, had bought the motion picture rights and formed his own company to make it. American actor John Garfield was slated to come to Beijing to play the lead. But before bringing over the cast, Howe wanted to shoot some preliminary footage. Or, as he said in his best Beverly Hills slang, "First we gotta get somethin' in the can."

Sometimes I think the denizens of Hollywood view the whole world as one big movie set. They don't care what real-life dramas might be unfolding around them, as long as the local atmosphere and background scenery fit their needs. In any case, Jimmy, as everybody called him, appeared script in hand in Beijing, oblivious to the fact that the city was already doomed. He didn't seem to realize that there was no chance of his finishing the film before Beijing fell.

Another problem he faced was the fact that, by 1948, most of the rickshaws in Beijing had already been replaced by pedicabs. There was one more minor difficulty. Howe, the celebrated cameraman known for filming such hits as *Kings Row* and *Abe Lincoln in Illinois,* didn't speak Mandarin or any other Chinese dialect. His father had worked as a coolie on the construction of the Northern Pacific Railway and brought Jimmy to the U.S. when he was only five.

For one scene in the movie Jimmy succeeded in rounding up some fifty rickshaw boys who were still using the old human-drawn conveyances. He ordered them to line up in front of the Grand Hotel des Wagon-Lits, presumably waiting for fares. That was fine for the still pictures Birns was shooting for our *Life* story about the making of this movie. But Jimmy wanted action. "Chop chop! Run run!" he kept shouting to the army of extras standing motionless beside their rickshaws in front of the hotel. "I'm paying you sonsabitches by the hour. Chop chop! Run run!"

Well, the rickshaw boys stood their ground. They couldn't understand why this Chinese man didn't address them in their native tongue. But they weren't stupid. "No run with empty rickshaw," explained the hotel doorman, who was decked out for the movie in a uniform with more gold braid than a Chinese admiral's.

Before John Garfield and the rest of the cast ever got to Beijing, General Fu Zuoyi decided to sue for peace. But he wasn't certain how or when to proceed. His ambivalence was well-known. Sitting in his Winter Palace headquarters, still uncertain of Mao's strategy, he was said to have changed his mind nine or ten times. Were the Communist armies going to sweep south into central China and attack Nanjing and Shanghai? Or were they going to attack Beijing and Tianjin? He still didn't know.

But Fu did know the significance of Beijing to Mao. It was there the Communist leader had come as a country boy from Hunan to learn about Marxism. The city also had strong links with China's past that Mao knew and cherished: how two thousand years ago it was a tiny garrison called Qi, soon to be wiped out by the first emperor, Qin Shi Huangdi. Then how under the Han Dynasty it became known as Yanjing, before the great Mongol emperor, Kublai Khan, in 1276 made it his capital, which Marco Polo called Khanbaliq. And, finally, how in 1664 the Manchus took over the city and renamed it Beijing (northern capital). That long and eventful history made Beijing an unmistakable symbol of power to Mao.

The long-awaited "siege of Beijing," as it was called, began on December 13, 1948, but consisted of only a couple of sporadic sorties. By that time, Birns and I had given up hope of ever seeing Fu and had gone south to rejoin Chiang's armies defending the Yangtze Valley. Later, we learned that the few heavy artillery rounds the Communists did pump into Beijing turned out to be duds. According to accounts published after the war, the Communists admitted to using non-exploding shells simply as a scare tactic. But then, the soldiers on both sides knew Mao wanted Beijing taken intact so he could make it his capital. As a result, they simply stood their watch and cursed the cold wind sweeping down from Inner Mongolia.

With General Lin Biao's troops still poised for attack, Mao's agents were already in touch with members of Fu's staff trying to agree on the rough terms of surrender. Perhaps even more important, as was also revealed after the war, Communist agents in Tianjin had succeeded in recruiting Fu's daughter, Fu Dongju, providing Lin Biao with a family member as an intermediary. When her father refused to capitulate, Mao joked about Fu holding out for ten more catties of pork. (One catty equals one pound-and-a-third.)

Down in Nanjing, the generalissimo steadfastly opposed Beijing's surrender even though his vice president, Li Zongren, urged Fu to sue for peace and had dispatched the former mayor of Beijing to negotiate with the Communists. But the man was assassinated by Chiang's secret police before he got there.

As one of the most trusted Nationalist commanders, Fu still felt a certain loyalty to the generalissimo even though they had never been close personally. "I will defend this city to the last," he proclaimed in what appeared to be yet another change of mind. And for a brief time he made it look as if he intended to do so. But the Communists became impatient, branding him a major war criminal, while at the same time offering him a pardon if he surrendered.

Astutely, the Red propagandists also began broadcasting promises directly to the people, describing how they and their property would be protected. "Except for a few major war criminals and notorious reactionaries," the Communists announced, "all Guomindang officials, police, and government members will be pardoned, provided they don't offer resistance."

Fu refused to budge even though the burden of supporting some 150,000 troops inside the city had become intolerable. When his soldiers had first started moving in, they occupied every palace and historic site, including the Temple of Heaven and Forbidden City. The late arrivals moved into schools and government buildings. But Fu's commanders made little attempt to care for the remaining troops, leaving them to fend for themselves. Soldiers roamed the streets knocking on doors. "We're moving in," they said, brushing the occupants aside.

Food supplies were also dwindling. Making things worse, the Communists had captured the Shihchingshan power plant fifteen miles southwest of Beijing. At first they shut down the city's electricity completely, then only partially, forcing the people to grope through dark streets and light their homes with kerosene lanterns. The city's water supply, dependent on electric pumps, also failed periodically. People gave up bathing and lined up at municipal wells for their drinking water. A strict 8:00 P.M. curfew was imposed, and a discipline supervisory corps was established to combat looting, currency speculation, rumormongering, and anything else that might create social unrest. Trucks carrying police wielding submachine guns and huge broad-blade swords careened through the streets, threatening on-the-spot executions of any troublemakers.

Amidst this chaos, the military authorities concentrated on bulldozing two new airstrips inside Beijing's walls. Soldiers, together with hordes of civilian laborers forced to work without pay, chopped down trees and telephone poles on the landing field approaches, while scavengers dashed out to gather up the pieces for firewood. In just four days, the former polo field near the old legation quarter had been turned into an improvised airport. A second airstrip next to the Temple of Heaven was also quickly completed. But after the first two Nationalist air force planes landed, it was discovered that both cramped landing fields were too short for the planes to take off, serving only as one-way streets into Beijing until they were lengthened.

Even with the renewed air link to Nanjing and Shanghai, the arriving planes brought little food and few medicines, but, to the dismay of the hungry populace, unlimited cartons of smuggled cigarettes. The pilots found cigarette cartons wedged in the wheel wells, hidden under the elevator cables, and stashed in nooks and crannies where they could have caused the planes to crash if left undetected. The departing planes, on the other hand, were packed with people, mostly fleeing businessmen and government officials.

The CAT pilots flying out of Beijing likened the crudely hacked-out airstrips to ripe camembert, not only because they were ripe for a fall to the Communists, but the bumpy take-offs caused most of the passengers to throw up. "First one would puke, and then they'd all puke in a chorus of vomiting," recalled Captain Felix Smith. "The smell of vomit in the cabin was so bad that after landing in Shanghai, we'd climb out the cockpit window, walk back along the top of the airplane, and jump off the tail."

Suddenly, for no apparent reason at all, feverish defense preparations started to be made again. Trenches and foxholes were dug and pillboxes and barricades erected at the main intersections, as if saving Beijing might come down to hand-to-hand fighting in the streets. "Is Fu trying to increase his bargaining power with the Communists?" some citizens asked. "He's holding us hostage," others complained.

General Lin Biao responded by broadcasting an ultimatum directly to the people. "You are completely surrounded. Your way of retreat has been completely cut off. There is only one course of action for you, and that is to surrender en masse. If you do not kill our soldiers who are prisoners and hand over all your weapons and industrial plants intact, we will treat you generously. As for Fu Zuoyi, although he has been listed as a war criminal, we will give him another chance to repent."

Still, Fu didn't feel that he personally could speak out in favor of a peaceful settlement. In his eyes, that would have made him a traitor to Chiang. But his secret representatives could. The first to do so was Liang Shuming, an old scholar and politician who had long advocated making Beijing an open city. Yenching University Professor of Philosophy Chang Tung-sun quickly joined him. Soon, members of the city council and other government officials added their voices to the clamor for peace. Student groups also became more assertive in demanding an end to the military standoff, although peace mongering, as well as rumormongering, was still a criminal offense. However vague, those peace overtures were welcomed by the people as good omens.

The astrological signs were also good—and in China that was always important. According to the so-called Yellow Calendar, 1948 was the Year of the Rat, and the month of December came in the eleventh moon. The people of Beijing, who put great faith in those things, remembered that "If the sun was shining on the day of Tung Chih (December 22), the people next year would be singing peaceful songs." The siege had not yet ended. But the day of Tung Chih dawned sunny and bright.

Mao, who by then was focusing his attention on the big battle looming for control of Nanjing and Shanghai, left the serious peace negotiations to what the people of Beijing dubbed "the Communist odd couple"—the smoothly diplomatic Zhou Enlai, together with the menacing tough guy Lin Biao. Although the two were bitter rivals in vying for Mao's favor, they were both against taking Beijing by force. After a series of meetings between them and Fu's representatives, a tentative peace agreement was reached.

Still, General Fu Zuoyi never publicly revealed his intentions. Without warning, on January 22, 1949, his headquarters simply announced the signing of an agreement designed "to shorten the civil war and to satisfy the public desire for peace . . . and prevent the vitality of the country from shrinking any further." The agreement made no mention of surrender. But it provided for Fu's twenty-five remaining divisions to be absorbed into the Red Army. Officers and enlisted men were permitted to retain their ranks, while those choosing to return to civilian life were given three months' pay and sent home. Beijing, thereby, became the first city in the civil war to come under Communist control through peaceful negotiation. It was also a face-saving solution for General Fu, who, it was said, "obeyed the siren song for peace sung by Zhou Enlai," before disappearing.

The news of Fu's ultimate surrender was frustrating for Birns and me. We had wasted several weeks pursuing the vaunted Nationalist general, who vanished without a trace. "Where's Fu?" our editors cabled, assuming he must have fled to Nanjing, where he could still be interviewed for a *Life* profile. "Fu who," I felt like replying, but restrained myself.

A few years later, in a stunning postwar resurrection, Fu Zuoyi reappeared in Beijing as Mao Zedong's minister of water conservancy.

10

THE MILLION-MAN BATTLE

As one Nationalist minister put it, "Manchuria is a limb that has been amputated. The body can live despite amputation. North China is another limb, and even it has been sacrificed. But central China is the Nationalist heart. And if the heart is pierced, the body dies."

That simply was a more poetic way of saying that the fate of Nationalist China didn't hinge on Chiang Kai-shek holding Mukden, Taiyuan, or Beijing. Rather, it was about to be decided In the dusty old market town of Xuzhou, where the Grand Canal bisects the Yellow River Plain in the heart of China.

Mao Zedong was now trying to pierce that heart. To deliver the fatal blow, he had amassed two powerful Communist columns pointing like twin daggers at the rail hub of Xuzhou. Pronounced "shoe Joe," the nondescript little city of 300,000 straddled the north-south Tianjin–Nanjing railroad line and the east-west Lunghai line in Jiangsu Province. In that key position, it was the gateway to Nanjing, the Nationalist capital, and to the great commercial metropolis of Shanghai. If Xuzhou fell, so, almost surely, would the rest of Chiang's China. That was the prediction of almost every reporter covering the war.

In field orders issued on October 11, 1948, the Communist leader called on his troop commanders to "complete the campaign on the plain surrounding Xuzhou in November and December." Then, he added sensibly, "Rest and consolidate your forces in January before crossing the Yangtze."

In Manchuria, Mao had already switched from guerrilla warfare to fighting conventional battles with massed armies. Now, sweeping in from my old CNRRA stomping grounds around Kaifeng, two hundred miles to the west, came the One-Eyed Dragon, Liu Bocheng, with 400,000 Communist troops. From the northeast, in neighboring Shandong Province, came the hard-bitten poet-general Chen Yi, commander in chief of the Communists' East China Theater, with another 200,000 men. A third Communist force led by General Chen Keng provided support. The whole area seethed with Red forces on the move.

These fighting units were aided by a civilian army of laborers numbering some two million men and women, mobilized by the young Communist Party leader, Deng Xiaoping. He conscripted peasants the same way the Nationalists had done, imposing stiff quotas for each village and threatening severe penalties if those quotas weren't met. During the battle, which raged for more than two months, Deng's army of farmers carried stores and ammunition, dug trenches and tank traps, and conducted a vicious anti-Nationalist propaganda campaign in the surrounding villages. Their activities were aimed at eliminating the tactical advantage of the Nationalist forces that entered the fray with tanks and planes.

Chiang Kai-shek recognized that his own survival depended on the outcome of this crucial battle. He held nothing back, committing fifty-five divisions, totaling 600,000 men, a force exactly matching the Communists'. Among them was his treasured tank corps, commanded by his second son, Chiang Weigo.

Gambling on fall floods to help him defend the swampy plain to the north and northwest, the generalissimo concentrated his armies east of Xuzhou City. He guessed right. The Communists attacked from the east and the Nationalists were there to meet the assault in the greatest battle in China's history—and the biggest fought anywhere since World War II.

After two weeks of bitter fighting, both sides were in a precarious position. Cloudless days and nights with a bright moon had helped the Nationalist air force disrupt the Communist supply lines, as Generals Liu Bocheng and Chen Yi tried to reinforce their badly mauled forces. At the same time, Chiang's Seventh Army Group, commanded by Lieutenant General Huang Botao, had been cut off and was being pummeled by Red mortars and artillery.

At this critical moment, *Life* photographer Birns, *Time* correspondent Robert Doyle, and I decided to fly north from Nanjing to cover what Chiang and his Nationalist generals called the Battle of Xuzhou. Mao and his followers, who later would brag to American visitors that this was China's Gettysburg, referred to it as the Battle of the Huai-Hai (after the muddy Huai River to the south, and the first syllable of Haizhou, a rail terminus to the east). By any name, emperors and warlords had considered the pivotal fights for this one small part of China as the climax accompanying every change of dynasty. Mao, obviously, viewed it the same way.

Landing in a Chinese air force transport, we found Xuzhou overwhelmed with refugees and soldiers. Fortunately, though, it had not been hit with the panic of a mass exodus that had paralyzed Mukden. The city was packed, but calm. Thousands of coolies, collected at random from the teeming streets, were digging trenches and patching the city's thick protective wall.

Trucks and ambulances filled with wounded soldiers rumbled in from the front, twenty-five miles to the east. More wounded arrived heaped high in mule carts, while the most seriously injured followed in rickshaws or suspended from bamboo poles shouldered by sweating bearers. At the French Canadian Catholic mission, where I had stayed occasionally while rounding up stray railway cars for CNRRA, I was told that Brother Kollar, the cook, was as usual, performing makeshift surgery on the wounded. I remembered how he used to say that those operations done on the kitchen table reminded him of a passage from a book by O. S. Marden: "Such stupidity!

The real surgeons are handling the meat saws and cleavers, while the butchers amputate human limbs."

The Nationalists' Thirteenth Army Group was still grimly defending Xuzhou. Word had gotten through to Lieutenant General Li Mi that the *Time* and *Life* team was coming, and he had sent his adjutant to meet us at the airstrip. The red-cheeked adjutant spotted us watching a couple of P-51 Mustangs being loaded with bombs for their next sortie. "We go see general," he said, proudly displaying his English. "She very busy today," he added, also demonstrating that he, like so many Chinese, had a gender problem with our language.

Heading out in the adjutant's jeep, we were escorted by a truck mounted with Bren guns. The two vehicles churned the fine dust into a brown cloud that clung to the road behind us. It was slow going. Stretching ahead to the horizon tramped some 25,000 men of the Seventy-second Army Group. "Help-out soldiers," the adjutant called them. Evidently, they were heading for the front to reinforce Li Mi's Thirteenth Army Group.

In addition to their rifles and backpacks, the soldiers carried huge cooking pots and coils of telephone wire as they marched doggedly toward the thump of artillery and crunch of bombs. Far ahead to the east and in some of the rocky hills to the south, we could see puffs of white billowing from where the shells and bombs found their targets.

We passed through a village that the adjutant explained had been retaken the day before. About all the Communists had left behind were slogans splashed in white paint across the mud walls of the burned-out houses: FIGHT ON TO NANJING! CAPTURE THE LIAR CHIANG ALIVE!" An old woman squatting in front of one of the gutted houses whacked at her laundry with a wooden paddle, oblivious to these exhortations or to the shelling, which was getting louder.

The bodies of a few Communist soldiers lay rotting by the roadside. From their dirty uniforms and frozen gray features, it was hard to tell them from the Nationalists marching past us. Bob Doyle noticed that one of the dead soldiers had what appeared to be a wound from a pistol shot in the back of his head. "Was that man executed?" he asked the adjutant. The adjutant didn't answer, but it was obvious that there were not enough medical facilities to care even for the wounded Nationalists.

A procession of mules hauling captured Communist rifles and machine guns passed through the village. Among the war booty, I spotted some old American Enfields and a few Japanese rifles that I couldn't identify. "Belong *Ba Lu*," explained the adjutant, indicating that the weapons had been lost on the battlefield by soldiers from Liu Bocheng's Eighth Route Army.

The adjutant pointed toward a hill where General Li Mi was directing artillery fire. Our jeep veered off the road, following a telephone wire stretched across the parched, lumpy land already sown with winter wheat. On top of the hill, we shook hands with the handsome general. About a hundred soldiers sprawled over the steep, craggy slope eating their evening bowls of rice. Tommy guns and rifles rested across their laps or on the slope behind them. Some read old newspapers while they ate. Others gazed absently over the rich brown, furrowed plain presently held by the 50,000 troops of their Thirteenth Army Group.

"Come sit on my sofa," said the general, motioning to a rock ledge. Li Mi, we knew, had learned English while serving under General Stilwell in Burma, now called Myanmar. There, he had also earned the reputation for being a good leader and hard fighter. A deep scar creased his left cheek. "My Burma decoration," he called it.

An orderly brought yellow pears that were as big as grapefruits. As we munched on the pears, Li traced the battle lines on the palm of his hand. Twelve miles to the east, his old comrade, Lieutenant General Huang Botao, and his Seventh Army Group, were encircled. They were trapped in the railway town of Nienchuang, Li explained, an area only three miles in diameter. Huang, he claimed, had already lost 40,000 men in eleven days defending that shrinking perimeter.

Li, from his position above the rail line, was driving south and east, attempting to relieve Huang. At the same time, the Nationalists' Second Army Group, commanded by General Chui Ching-chuan, was pushing up from the other side of the rail line. "We have orders from the generalissimo to advance at any cost," said Li. "In eight days we have gone eight miles. But this is the worst fighting I have ever experienced. I've lost two hundred officers and more than eight thousand soldiers."

As Li continued to brief us, a Chinese air force Mustang hummed along in the fading twilight and then swooped down on a village about three miles to the east. We could hear the chatter of machine guns. "That village is Makutze," said Li. "It's my objective tonight. After the sun sets, my artillery will open up and then the infantry will move in."

The glowing red sun dropped below the horizon, and a white ground mist crawled slowly up the valley floor, covering the black line of the Lung-hai railroad. Lights from the Chia Wang coal mine, captured by the Communists ten days earlier, twinkled brightly ten miles to the north. Li's adjutant cranked the field phone and shouted curt commands to the forward gun positions. Suddenly, the war was on.

Huge muzzle flashes from 105mm howitzers ballooned from the plain, hung for an instant, and then blinked out. Ahead of the artillery, the 37mm guns on Li's tanks cut red streaks through the blackness. Occasional flares and signal lights lit up the sky. Between the thundering blasts came the incongruous creak and groan of an oxcart bumping its way across the field below. After an hour, the barrage slowed and flames licked the sky over Makutze. "Now come the infantry," said Li, who also indicated it was time for dinner.

Our jeep trailed behind the general's as we ground in low gear across the rough fields towards his headquarters in Zhouzhuang village, near the front. The two drivers kept flicking their lights on and off trying to skirt the deeper holes. The bumpy ride reminded me that it was just a year since I had stopped making those bone-rattling runs for CNRRA over neighboring Henan Province's rutted roads. There, my truck convoys had faced threats from the same two Communist generals fighting here, Liu Bocheng and Chen Yi.

As we neared General Li's headquarters, we passed an artillery position. The hulking forms of tanks also loomed up against the night sky. A 105mm gun directly in front of the tanks cut loose, its red flash silhouetting for an instant the crouched figures of its gun crew. The acrid smell of gunpowder wafted over our jeeps. Li leaned out and said in Chinese, "Careful, careful, we are passing under your muzzle."

The Thirteenth Army Group headquarters was located in a small compound ringed by freshly dug trenches. Mud pillboxes bristled with machine guns, and sentries lurked in every doorway. Outside the door of the general's hut, a soldier squatted beside a twig fire drying his cotton shoes. Inside the hut, one of Li's officers was bent over a map. Two candles stuck upright in their own wax drippings on the table provided the only light. In the corner of the room were a cot and a couple of benches.

Li motioned for us to pull up the benches and sit down as he called for food. Orderlies quickly appeared with steaming dishes of chicken, bean sprouts, and pork—remarkably, ten courses in all. Nevertheless, with typical Chinese politeness, the general apologized for not serving rice wine.

The periodic booming of Li's artillery punctuated the meal. Once, the general was called to the phone. He talked for a moment in a low voice and then returned to the table. In the candlelight, the·lines of his youthful face sagged. He stared at his rice bowl and then explained that he had just received a radio message from his friend General Huang Botao. "The Communist trap is closing," said Li. "We must reach him in two days."

After dinner he led us across the compound to another hut, where we were to spend the night. Through the bright moonlight, Chinese air force planes droned overhead, some dropping bombs that shook the ground, others, as Li explained, silently parachuting supplies to the encircled General Huang.

Again, Li apologized—this time for our crude quarters and for the straw-covered boards that were our beds. But sleep was out of the question. The howitzers dug in behind the village, kept up their intermittent fire. First came the muzzle blast, then the scream of the shell overhead, finally the distant crunch as the shell exploded. Added to those sounds was the throbbing pulse beating in my ears. For a couple of days I had felt sick, with a low-grade fever coming on late each afternoon. Now, I could feel the fever rising. My forehead was wet with sweat.

Shortly before midnight, the crackle of small-arms fire seemed to be drawing closer. Li Mi had shown us a pillbox just outside the door of our hut where we were to take cover if the Communists counterattacked. "Don't try to leave the compound," he warned us. "You'll run right into our own machine gun fire."

When we met Li, I noticed he was wearing a private's uniform. At dinner, he told us that he also wore fake dog tags bearing the name Li Wen-hua, the Chinese equivalent of John Smith, in case he was captured. Very smart, I thought. But with the rifle fire sounding dangerously close, those precautions of his didn't exactly bolster my confidence that his troops would be able to hold. So I reached over and woke the adjutant who was bedded down next to me and asked if the time had come to seek refuge in the pillbox. He roared with laughter. *"Buyaojin, buyaojin"* ("no matter, no matter"), he said in Chinese. Then, remembering that I was an American, he added, "No worry. Same thing every night. Communists attack. But we stop."

He was right. Glancing outside at first light, everything looked the same. Soldiers carrying bowls of steaming rice ambled along the narrow streets of the village. Now I could see the streets had been carved into a network of trenches and foxholes. Li's troops were dug in everywhere. Mortar and machine gun emplacements occupied the heart of the village, while tanks and howitzers were parked on the fringes just beyond the dilapidated village wall. But amid all this modern equipment were signs of China's ancient past. A donkey hitched to a centuries-old wooden-wheeled cart loaded with shining 105mm shell cases slowly munched hay outside of our hut.

In just twenty-four hours, Li's troops had transformed this peaceful village into a bristling fortress. Most of the residents had fled. Those remaining puttered dazedly around their mud huts. A few timidly crept up to the soldiers knotted around the army's steaming rice cauldrons in hopes of getting some food. Freshly painted Nationalist slogans splashed over the mud walls exhorted, SOLDIERS AND CIVILIANS COOPERATE TO EXTERMINATE THE RED BANDITS.

Inside Li's headquarters hut we found the general splashing water on his face from a tin basin. His adjutant reported that he had a good night until three A.M. But over breakfast the general explained that his troops had been unable to capture Makutze. Although a thousand shells had been poured into the village, the Communists held their line and mustered enough strength to send a counterattack within half a mile of Li's headquarters. "We will take Makutze today," he said confidently. "We must. We attack at ten."

We wanted to go back with Li to his hilltop artillery observation post to watch the battle as it progressed. The odds didn't seem very good for rescuing General Huang Botao. Yet Li's courage and determination were convincing. The compassion he showed for his cornered comrade-in-arms was touching. Li Mi was certainly different from any Nationalist general I had met before. From the moment we arrived, I noticed the deep concern he showed for his soldiers.

By nine o'clock, my fever was still rising. According to Birns, the whites of my eyes were turning yellow. A number of the CAT pilots we had flown with recently had come down with jaundice, and I suspected that might be my problem.

"I'm afraid I must return to Shanghai," I told the general. He had enough worries, so I didn't mention my fever. When Birns and Doyle announced they were going too, Li seemed genuinely disappointed that none of us would be there to watch the artillery bombardment and, following it, the infantry assault on Makutze.

Returning to Xuzhou, we boarded a Chinese air force C-46 that was going to parachute ammunition into Nienchuang, where General Huang's Seventh Army Group was surrounded. After that, the plane would fly straight to Nanjing, and from there we could hitch another ride to Shanghai.

As the C-46 spiraled down to 2,000 feet over Nienchuang, we saw crumpled parachutes from previous drops covering the brown ground all around General Huang's headquarters. From the air we also got a good view of the town's heart-shaped double wall and double moat nestled up against the smashed Lunghai railway. Trenches webbed out from the outer wall like some scabrous disease infecting the good earth. We could see corpses and shattered artillery pieces dotting the trenches. The southern section of the town was burning, and pillars of smoke rose from all the nearby villages as well.

The Nationalists still enjoyed unchallenged command of the air, and Chinese P-51 Mustangs and B-24 bombers were pounding the open fields surrounding Nienchuang, where the Communists were dug in.

Our C-46 began to drop its cargo. Communist guns outside Nienchuang opened fire on our plane, and puffs of black smoke blossomed all around us in the sky. Fortunately, the antiaircraft gunners were short of their mark.

The day after we returned to Shanghai, word came that Nienchuang's moated walls had been pierced. General Huang Botao was reported by the Communists to have committed suicide while his segmented army was being chewed to pieces by Communist poet and strategist General Chen Yi. After the war, when he became China's foreign minister, Chen summed up this victory with a verse:

> *When old friends meet and inquire about me,*
> *tell them to look closely at the desolation in the*
> *enemy's rear.*

Of course, that wasn't the way the government reported the situation. "The enemy offensive has suffered a complete collapse," claimed the Central News Agency. "Because of the continued pressure of the Nationalist forces, the Communists are having to fight like cornered animals to avoid annihilation." But it was Li Mi's troops who were fighting like cornered animals. Having seriously overextended their lines trying to rescue General Huang, they had left themselves open to a calamitous pincer attack.

We were lucky to have gotten out when we did. Suddenly, all the evacuation planes were crammed with soldiers "dying in their blood and excrement on the flights back to Shanghai," as CAT Captain Felix Smith described the round-the-clock rescue missions he flew from Xuzhou. "I landed at Shanghai's Hungjao Airport after midnight hoping for, but not expecting, military ambulances," he wrote in *China Pilot.* "There were none. Our airline laborers carried the stretchers to a grassy plot beside the tarmac where our own doctors and nurses, using flashlights, examined them. Some soldiers moaned. Some cried for water. Others were silent, which seemed even worse."

The initial report on my own physical condition wasn't much cheerier, though, unfortunately, it proved to be accurate. I was diagnosed as having typhoid fever and hepatitis, a debilitating combination that kept me in the hospital for four weeks.

During my confinement, the battle for Xuzhou raged on, but with no reprieve for Chiang's troops. Stuck in bed, I reflected on the generalissimo's rapidly failing leadership. Even *Time,* ordinarily pro-Chiang Kai-shek, reported that his "prestige has sunk lower than the Yangtze." The magazine quoted an American observer as saying, "The generalissimo's name is now mud among all classes."

Yet, at sixty-one, the besieged president remained uncompromising. He continued to portray himself as China's salvation. And, as the heir to Sun Yat-sen, the republic's founder, he kept on publicly repeating Sun's Three Principles: *Min Tsu* ("national unity"), *Min Chuan* ("political democracy"), and *Min Sheng* ("people's livelihood"). Chiang also bade his field commanders to remember Sun's dying words: "You shall never yield to the enemy."

Nevertheless, Chiang failed to see that the feudalism which Sun had fought to eradicate still flourished, just as he seemed blind to the fact that, by outlawing even the most innocuous liberal movements, he was driving their members over to the Communists.

On the battlefield, defections were also jeopardizing his key defensive maneuvers. Yet, when the Communists switched from guerrilla warfare to fighting conventional battles with massed armies, as they had done at Mukden and now Xuzhou, Chiang claimed he welcomed the change in their tactics. His air force and armored corps, he declared, would at last give him the edge.

Buoyantly, he popped in and out of his private map room, masterminding his troop commanders' movements by long-distance telephone. But, as Li Mi had hinted, the generalissimo was interfering too much. His daily calls from Nanjing failed to take into account developments at the front. Even worse, he became furious with his generals' defeats—and, in some cases, defections—claiming, "They think only of their own positions and nothing of the country they are supposed to defend."

Mao, on the other hand, in a statement made to Xinhua, the Communist news agency, proclaimed that "the military situation has reached a turning point and the balance of forces between the two sides has undergone a fundamental change. The People's Liberation Army troops, long superior in quality, have become superior in numbers as well." He characterized the Nationalist defenses as "collapsing like a soft wall."

After sixty-five days of fierce fighting at Xuzhou, Chiang's forces were defeated. Of the Nationalist divisions, 550,000 men had been lost. More than 300,000 of them were captured, including most of his son's vaunted armored corps. The rest either died or defected. General Tu Yu-ming, Chiang's deputy field commander, changed into a dead Communist soldier's uniform and pretended to be a prisoner of his own aide-de-camp, but the ruse failed, and Tu also was captured. The Communists claimed Nationalist supplies were so short that Tu's last meal before being captured was his American sheepskin-lined gloves.

Li Mi, I was glad to learn while I was still recovering in the hospital, managed to elude the enemy. Two years later, he showed up in northern Myanmar, and from there continued to lead forays against Communist garrisons in China's border province of Yunnan.

How he escaped from the Xuzhou battlefield was widely disputed. Some said he flew away with Chiang Weigo, the generalissimo's son. Others claimed he was taken prisoner, but broke out of a Communist jail. Still others reported that he disguised himself as a merchant and was hauled through Communist lines in a wheelbarrow. The most likely story, though, was that he and remnants of his Thirteenth Army Group, trudged all the way to a base in Myamar's mountainous Shan States, which Li remembered from his World War II days with Stilwell.

What happened to Li Mi's anti-Communist fighters after that has been well documented. Soon, unmarked C-46s were flying in weapons to him in Myanmar, purchased by wealthy Chinese merchants in Bangkok. For a while, even the U.S. was secretly airlifting arms to Li's strike force for their hit-and-run attacks inside China. Myanmar was too busy combating its own rebels to pester Li. But, after he built his group of 1,700 ragtag fighters into the powerful 10,000-man National Salvation Army, as he named it, the Myanmar government complained to the United Nations.

A heart attack finally forced Li to leave Myanmar in 1953. But, by then, many of his soldiers had married local girls and taken up farming. That made it easier for William "Wild Bill" Donovan, the former U.S. spy chief who was then Ambassador to Thailand, to negotiate a deal to fly the National Salvation Army's 2,000 die-hards to Taiwan, where General Li Mi had also retired.

For the rest of Chiang's troops who fought at Xuzhou, the battle ended horribly. Horses were slaughtered for food. The surrounded Nationalist soldiers began peeling bark from the trees and scrounging for roots in the fields. They were even reduced to clipping up coffins to burn as firewood. Women and children froze to death in crowded huts. On the edge of the city, Communist loudspeakers offered food and safety if the Nationalists would surrender. "There is no escape," the loudspeakers boomed before the final artillery barrage began.

Even Mao's hard-bitten troops were shocked by the devastation they found in Xuzhou: "Belsen-like open graves into which hundreds of human carcasses had been tossed" and "a ghostly hospital where the patients were all found dead in their beds," according to an article in the Communist magazine, *Red Flags Flying*. It reported that the first Communist patrols probing the narrow streets of the old city, were forced to don gas masks because "they couldn't stand the stench of the putrifying flesh, although the surviving residents seemed not to notice it."

As usual, the Central News Agency refused to call the debacle a defeat. "No longer of strategic importance, Xuzhou has been evacuated," it claimed.

Just before the Nationalists surrendered on January 10, 1949, Chiang Kai-shek dispatched his wife to the U.S. once again to lobby Congress and the American public for emergency support. Chiang also sent another desperate appeal for help to President Truman. But Major General Barr, head of the Joint U.S. Military Advisory Group In China, known by its acronym, MAGIC ("using magic," its officers facetiously said, "was the only way Chiang could still win"), had already convinced Truman of the futility of sending more military aid. "No battle has been lost since my arrival due to a lack of ammunition or equipment," Barr cabled the president. "The Nationalists' military debacles, in my opinion, can all be attributed to the world's worst leadership and other morale-destroying factors which led to a complete loss of the will to fight."

Several months earlier, Barr had advised Chiang to concede Manchuria to the Communists and concentrate his troops south of the Yellow River. The generalissimo was aghast at the proposal, notifying Truman that in no way could he be induced to follow Barr's suggestion. Now, after the rout of his armies in Xuzhou, Chiang stood in imminent danger of losing what the Chinese called the "Mandate of Heaven"—the support of his own followers. According to the ancient warning delivered to the ruling princes by the philosopher Mencius, "Heaven hears as the people hear; Heaven sees as the people see." And the Nationalists were hearing and seeing defeat wherever they looked.

Truman himself could no longer abide the generalissimo and expressed his feelings in an angry letter to a friend: "Chiang Kai-shek's downfall was his own doing. His generals surrendered the equipment we gave him to the Commies, who then used the arms and ammunition to destroy him." That, however, was not true in the battle for Xuzhou, where many of the Nationalists had fought bravely and died. To his scolding remarks, Truman added: "Only an American army of two million men could have saved the generalissimo, and that would have been World War III."

Mao Zedong, although welcoming the outcome of the Battle of the Huai-Hai, as he called it, now worried about how to control and provide food for the hundred million people living in the greatly expanded territory behind Communist lines. "Could the peasants of the Central Plain be expected to begin sowing in the spring when so many of them had been mobilized for war?" he questioned his subordinates. After all, if the people couldn't feed themselves, the Communists might quickly lose the loyalty of those they had liberated. But that threat didn't materialize.

Years later, the Communists gave much of the credit for their great victory in the Battle of the Huai-Hai to the heroic party organizer they cited for mobilizing the two million peasants to provide logistical support for the soldiers. "His pick-and-shovel crews," the Communists claimed, "neutralized Chiang's armored corps by digging a ring of tank traps around Xuzhou."

This belatedly acclaimed hero, Deng Xiaoping, eventually succeeded Mao as China's paramount leader.

11

THE GIMO FLEES AND THE GOLD FOLLOWS

The Battle of the Huai-Hai was Chiang Kai-shek's Waterloo, and even he, the ever-proud gimo, recognized how crushing that defeat was. In desperation, he formed a new war cabinet, persuading Sun Fo, the liberal son of Sun Yat-sen, to become premier, as if a shakeup in the Nationalist bureaucracy could keep the Communist armies from spreading south like hot lava. Ludicrously, the Central News Agency's "frontline" dispatches kept right on repeating Chiang's favorite pronouncement: "The bandits are fleeing in disorder," while Mao's propagandists reciprocated by branding Chiang and his wife "running dogs of American imperialism."

"After all I've done for China," the generalissimo fumed when he learned that the Communists had put him at the top of a list of forty-five war criminals. "How can we talk to such people?" However, Vice President Li Zongren and most of his cabinet said they were prepared to talk peace with Mao's representatives.

Furious with the cabinet as well, Chiang drove out to Purple Mountain to visit the mausoleum of Sun Yat-sen. He would draw strength, he said, from being in the presence of his former mentor. Observers watched the slim uniformed figure wearing a military cape and leaning on a cane mount the white stone stairway. Before entering the tomb, Chiang removed his cape and handed it to an aid. Then, stepping inside he bowed three times before Sun Yat-sen's white marble statue. When he emerged, he walked slowly down the steps, saluting the thousands of soldiers standing in formation around the mausoleum.

That was Chiang's last troop review on the mainland. In a final plea, he asked the U.S., Britain, France, and the Soviet Union to intervene with Mao. Each separately refused, leaving the Nationalist leader physically drained and psychologically beaten. "With the hope that hostilities may be brought to an end, and the people's suffering relieved," he announced to a group of loyal supporters, "I have decided to retire."

The small reception room at the Ministry of Defense on that afternoon of January 21, 1949, was jammed with government officials. As usual, the generalissimo wore a simple khaki uniform without insignia. Those inside said he spoke without emotion, "as if he was delivering a routine message of no special significance." An hour later, I watched this "beaten man," as Seymour Topping of the Associated Press described him, leave the ministry wearing a long blue gown and black jacket, the traditional dress of a Chinese gentleman. It was a clear and unusually warm winter day as he stepped into his black Cadillac bearing "No. 1" on its license plates. He seemed deep in his own thoughts, oblivious to the crowd gathered outside the ministry.

Awaiting him at Nanjing's military airport was the twin-engined *Mei-Ling*, named after Madame Chiang, who at that moment was still in Washington fruitlessly trying to muster support for her husband. Or, as President Truman caustically remarked, "Looking for some handouts." Chiang said perfunctory good-byes to the officials gathered to see him off. Slowly he climbed aboard the plane, and pulled the door shut himself, then headed first for dinner at the lake resort of Hangzhou, and then on to his hometown of Fenghua. We journalists assumed the generalissimo was retiring with Confucian humility to spend the rest of his days as a country squire. Actually, Fenghua was to be but a temporary stop, while he feverishly prepared to relocate on the island redoubt of Taiwan.

The *Mei-Ling* thundered down the runway, climbed, and circled Purple Mountain, where the white stone of Sun Yat-sen's mausoleum reflected the fading daylight. Watching the plane disappear over the horizon, I was struck by the fact that only thirty-seven years had elapsed since Dr. Sun, the rebellious little physician from Hawaii who became Chiang's mentor, overthrew the Manchus and established the Chinese Republic. It was also just ten days since Xuzhou fell, thereby ending the epic Battle of the Huai-Hai.

Although Chiang had left Nanjing, his supporters felt there was considerable ambiguity surrounding his retirement; that his departure did not represent final abdication and that he soon expected to be recalled as president. In fact, when Vice President Li Zongren arrived at the presidential palace to take over the reins of government, he was stunned to find that Chiang had named him "acting president," indicating it might be a temporary appointment. The generalissimo's written statement left for Li didn't include a word about retiring. Rather, it conveyed the impression that Li was merely to manage the affairs of state in his absence. Chiang also made it clear that he intended to remain head of the Guomindang Party.

Li refused to be intimidated. He brought a number of his old military pals from Guangxi Province and gave them impressive titles. He also kept in close touch with American Ambassador J. Leighton Stuart, giving the impression that, as acting president, he was in control. But Li's appeal for a $1 billion currency stabilization loan from the U.S. was ignored. Stuart recognized that it was far too late to rescue China's ravaged economy.

In many respects, rampant inflation and currency devaluation had eroded Chiang's public support more than the battlefield defeats. There is a saying in China: "Iron weighs as much as gold on the military scale." But as the Nationalist armies reeled back toward Nanjing and Shanghai, it was not just the tanks, cannons, and all the rest of the iron lost on the battlefield that hastened Chiang's resignation; the flight of gold and financial chaos that followed had further undermined his authority.

Beginning in August 1948, Chiang had tried to staunch the gold drain by imposing stringent currency reforms. It was a calculated, though desperate, gamble to impede a complete economic collapse. Everyone was ordered to surrender their gold, silver, and American greenbacks. In an unprecedented act of public faith, coins and pieces of precious metal were pulled from iron pots all over China and handed over to the government. New gold-backed bank notes called GY (gold yuan) were then issued in exchange.

At the same time, the generalissimo appointed Chiang Ching-kuo, his Russian-educated eldest son by his first marriage, to be economic czar of Shanghai. He hoped that if the chubby thirty-nine-year-old major general could make the reforms stick in Shanghai, where hoarding and speculation were rampant, he just might set an example for what was left of Nationalist China. First, Ching-kuo, as he was known, had to capture the city's attention, and he did this with a combination of scare tactics and humor.

Hauled through the streets in an open coffin appeared a grimacing corpse clutching a carton of cigarettes, two boxes of laundry soap, and a roll of cloth. Every block or two, the corpse would climb out of its coffin and harangue the crowd on the evils of hoarding and speculating. Signs painted on the coffin's two sides warned: THOSE WHO HOARD ARE PUBLIC ENEMIES. HE WHO DAMAGES THE GOLD YUAN WILL HAVE HIS HEAD CHOPPED OFF.

The generalissimo's son also attacked Shanghai's wealthy businessmen by branding them "armed robbers." He didn't care if they had given financial support to his father. "Their wealth and foreign-style homes," he railed, "are built on the skeletons of the people who live in crude sheds and cubbyholes, or writhe in the streets and ditches—a horde of beggars for whom wearing even a pair of grass sandals seems a rare luxury."

But then, Chiang Ching-kuo never did have much sympathy for *Dahu,* or "wealthy families." After graduating from Frunze Military Academy in Moscow, he worked on construction jobs in the Caucasus for nine years. "I had numberless hard days and did the lowest work," he told me. "But I survived thanks to my father's teaching that man's spirit, not his money, is omnipotent."

Returning to China with a blond Russian wife, he proved to be both tough and incorruptible in several apprentice posts in Jiangxi Province. He also demonstrated a strong anti-elitist philosophy and deep concern for the common man not shown by his father. So, in Shanghai it wasn't surprising when he shed his major general's uniform for an open-necked, short-sleeved shirt and listened like a good ward boss to people's complaints.

I went to one of those sessions. A laborer in black coolie pants was bewailing his boss's decision to close down his well-stocked rubber factory rather than sell his products at the new ceiling prices. Ching-kuo promised to investigate. He did, and the factory stayed open. He also met with the city's financiers, whom, he complained, are "friendly toward me in person. But behind my back there is no evil they won't commit."

At first, his get-tough measures seemed to be working. The banks closed for three days to convert the checking and savings accounts of their customers into gold yuan. When the banks reopened, they began exchanging the public's almost worthless old currency for GY at the rate of three million to one. Everybody appeared to cooperate with surprising good grace. I watched men and women stand in line for hours waiting to turn in whole suitcases and basket-loads of the crumpled old bills for crisp yellow-and-brown GY banknotes.

The new money, naturally, took getting used to. Until then, everybody in China was a millionaire. We Americans had become accustomed to arriving at a restaurant with a shopping bag full of cash to pay for dinner, or having an airline ticket invalidated right after it was purchased because the price of aviation fuel had doubled.

A few months earlier, I had written an article for *Life* on the Shanghai Telephone Company's hopelessly inflated six-billion-yuan fortnightly payroll. The story didn't run right away. By the time it was published, the company payroll had shot up to 385 billion yuan.

With the gold yuan everything changed. A trolley ticket cost only ten cents instead of 300,000 yuan, a copy of the *Shanghai Evening Post and Mercury* twenty-five cents instead of 750,000 yuan. Factory workers no longer had to sprint to the nearest rice shop each payday to beat the hourly price hikes. And a farmer could buy a water buffalo for fewer yuan than it formerly would have cost to feed the beast for a week.

To keep the value of the new currency from eroding, Ching-kuo enlisted hundreds of young volunteers from a paramilitary organization called the Bandit Suppression National Reconstruction Corps. They posted ceiling prices at all markets, raided warehouses looking for hoarded goods, and placed anonymous reporting boxes in the streets so consumers could squeal on the cheaters. During the first few weeks, several hundred merchants were arrested for overpricing.

"It doesn't matter if pork and perfume disappear from the markets," Chiang Kai-shek's son declared, "so long as the people aren't starving." However, he was only marginally concerned with small shopkeepers who added a few cents to a catty of pork or pack of cigarettes. It was the *Dalaohu,* or "big tigers," who were causing the commodity shortages and manipulating prices. "Traitorous merchants," he declared, "are disturbing the markets and deserve severe punishment." He soon acquired the reputation for being the fearless "big tiger hunter."

While most citizens had obediently turned in their gold and Amercian greenbacks, many of the wealthy families converted just enough to feign compliance. So Ching-kuo sent loudspeaker trucks out cruising the streets. They stopped in front of the homes of the rich, booming out orders to turn in their gold. The hoarders were further intimidated by claims that the loudspeaker trucks were equipped with special detection devices that could tell if precious metals were hidden in the houses. The chief suspects were then named in the newspapers.

Within days, a number of "big tigers," including members of some of the most famous families in Shanghai, were arrested. The story of Ching-kuo's crackdown was moving so fast it was difficult for us reporters to keep up with it. The son of the local gangster boss, "Big Ears" Du, one of the generalissimo's most powerful backers, was charged with illegal stock transactions after the Shanghai Stock Exchange had been shut down. The son of the celebrated Tiger Balm patent medicine king, Aw Boon Haw, was arrested for gold and foreign currency smuggling. But the story that drew worldwide attention, including *Life's,* was the execution of millionaire merchant and currency speculator Wang Chun-cheh, who was shot to death by a police executioner. The event caused a sensation in Shanghai. "In Wang's fine home," as I reported to the magazine, "his family cried out, but their tears made no impression on Chiang Ching-kuo, the man responsible for Wang's death. 'I would rather see one family cry,' he announced, 'than a whole street weeping.'"

Another well-publicized case, however, put a momentary brake on Ching-kuo's big tiger hunt. When word reached Madame Chiang that her nephew, David Kung, general manager of the Yangtze Development Corporation, was about to be arrested for hoarding, she stormed down to Shanghai to confront her stepson, with whom she'd always had a tempestuous relationship.

Right afterward, I tried to track down David and his sister Jeannette only to learn they had slipped away to Hong Kong. Their company subsequently moved its head office to Florida. But very few other big tigers escaped Ching-kuo's clutches. As Indian Ambassador K. M. Panikkar remarked,

> *For four weeks Shanghai was practically terror-stricken into good behavior. During that time prices held steady, although customers complained that meat sold at official prices had more bone, and that hens were apparently laying smaller eggs.*

Meanwhile, prices elsewhere in China kept right on rising. Shanghai was said to be a "tiny island of controlled prices in a raging sea of inflation." The more successful Ching-kuo was, the greater the pressure on Shanghai businessmen to sell their goods elsewhere, where prices continued to rise. For farmers, too, it made no sense to sell their produce in Shanghai when they could charge much more in other cities. Shanghai, therefore, began to experience desperate shortages of food and manufactured goods. This precipitated the expansion of Chiang Ching-kuo's jurisdiction to include Nanjing and three nearby provinces—Zhejiang, Jiangsu, and Anhui. But that move backfired. Restaurants emptied and medical supplies and other goods became unavailable. Everything simply vanished from store shelves, forcing the government to revoke the price controls altogether.

Ching-kuo promptly resigned and, accepting all the blame for "increasing the suffering of the people," publicly apologized for the failed economic reforms. "To make clear my responsibility," he said, "I am petitioning the government for my punishment." At the same time, he also expressed the hope that the people would "not again allow traitorous merchant-speculators, bureaucratic politicians, and ruffians and scoundrels to control Shanghai."

It quickly became evident that the whole economy was disintegrating. Food prices doubled each day, setting off rice riots in Shanghai as people demanded the return of price ceilings. Instead, the government banks began selling gold again, but for ten times what they paid for it when the new currency was issued. Even at that price, crowds stormed the banks to buy the precious metal. Seven people were trampled to death and forty-five injured in one Shanghai gold rush. But compared to the mountain of gold converted into the now virtually worthless GY, only a molehill was changed back. The rest remained secreted in sturdy wooden boxes in the vaults of three Shanghai banks.

One night strolling along the Bund near the Time–Life office, I found myself facing a detour. Several blocks had been cordoned off without explanation. Soldiers roamed the area with cocked pistols, guarding a fleet of trucks parked in front of the Central Bank of China. For the next five hours, a bucket brigade of coolies wearing special white armbands transferred hundreds of small, heavy crates from the bank to the trucks. At dawn, the trucks roared off to Jetty No. 12, where the crates were quickly stowed aboard the lighthouse tender *Hai Hsing*. Later, I learned that those wooden boxes contained seventy-five tons of gold. Another night, twenty-five more tons were removed from the Charter Bank and Bank of China and placed aboard a Chinese navy LST.

The government did its best to keep the massive gold transfer a secret. "The banks are moving their archives south," claimed the Central News

Agency. That obviously wasn't true, as the banks in Guangzhou, Shantou (Swatow) and Xiamen (Amoy) were also seen removing similar wooden crates from their vaults.

Bank vaults all along the China coast were also cleaned out of their silver bullion. The silver exodus might have been kept under wraps if it hadn't been for a shipping disaster in which 964 Chinese passengers were drowned. The death toll wasn't big news in China, accustomed to much worse catastrophes. But word leaked that the *Taiping*, which had collided with a coal barge and sunk eighty-five miles southeast of Shanghai, contained more than one hundred tons of silver. The lighthouse keeper on a nearby island let the secret out when he told the crew of an American LST that a Chinese Coast Guard vessel investigating the accident refused to leave any warning markers around the sunken ship for fear that pirates might attempt to salvage the silver.

By February 1, ten days after Chiang Kai-shek resigned as president, the news finally broke that a $300 million hoard of gold, and many more tons of silver, were safely tucked away in Taiwan—"the golden nest egg," as I called it in my report to *Life*, "that eventually financed the transplanted Nationalist government." At the same time, rumors (which later proved to be true) also surfaced that Madame Chiang Kai-shek, who was in Washington begging for support for China, had packed her trunks with gold bars, precious stones, and several million dollars in U.S. greenbacks, knowing that, as a VIP, arriving on an American navy plane, she wouldn't be subjected to a customs search.

Shanghai's speculators, grasping for whatever gold they could still find, turned to the pirates and smugglers of Macao. Every night, from the tiny Portuguese colony appended to the South China coast, a string of armed junks known as the "golden chain" slipped into Shanghai. Hidden in crevices under their teak deck planks were chunks of gold ranging in size from $22,000 ingots down to $50 slivers.

As Shanghai's demand for the yellow metal multiplied, so did the junks in the "golden chain." Jack Birns and I decided to fly down to Macao, figuring it would be a nice scoop for *Life* if we could trace those illegal shipments back to their source and discover who was behind the smuggling ring.

We arrived on a Catalina Flying Boat operated by Macao Air Transport, the same charter company that was hauling one planeload of gold after another into the Portuguese colony. Skimming across the jade green water of the *Porto Exterior,* our plane pulled up alongside another flying boat bobbing gently on the waves. We could see coolies wrestling wooden cases through its open hatch onto a launch. A police boat bristling with fifty-caliber machine guns patrolled back and forth. The boxes were smaller than beer cases, but extremely heavy. Each was plastered with more airline stickers than decorate a world traveler's suitcase. Labels marked Lima, Rio, Dakar, Amsterdam, Paris, Calcutta, and Saigon, traced the precious cargo's path around the globe.

There was nothing illegal about bringing gold into Macao. Portugal hadn't signed the Bretton Woods Monetary Agreement, which tied most nations to a fixed price for gold of thirty-five dollars an ounce. The crates entering Macao contained free-market gold sold to the highest bidder. And with the Chinese clamoring for more and more, a large portion of the world's free-market supply was being funneled into this minute, six-square-mile enclave—the spot where Europeans had obtained their first foothold in Asia four hundred years before.

We soon discovered that Macao's ruler, or dictator, was not the Portuguese governor, but a wiry little Malay-Chinese named Pedro Jose Lobo. He was born in East Timor, but raised in Macao by a Portuguese family. During World War II, he kept Macao alive by organizing a ring that smuggled food across the border from Japanese-occupied China. Eventually, he became head of the colony's Administrative Service Department, in charge of all imports, and in that position succeeded in levying two taxes on each ounce of gold arriving on the flying boats: an official tax of thirty-five cents for the Macao treasury, and another hidden tax of two dollars and ten cents for himself.

Lobo claimed to know nothing about Macao's "invisible export," as the gold smuggled to China was called. That $330-million-a-year business, we learned, was being handled by his silent partner, Ho Yin, owner of Macao's Tai Fong Bank.

It was easy enough locating Lobo, or "P. J.," as everybody called him. When he heard that a team from *Life* magazine was in Macao, he quickly found us. His hobby was composing, writing, staging, and conducting operettas, and he insisted on our photographing the opening night of his newest creation, *Cruel Separation*. But just finding Ho Yin, much less wangling our way into the bowels of his bank, where the gold bricks were secretly melted down, was another matter. Some people said the mercurial thirty-nine-year-old banker was in South Africa, others said South America. "Mr. Ho visits many countries buying gold," his secretary told us.

Jack and I were about to give up and fly back to Shanghai when a little man wearing black pajamas knocked on our hotel room door.

"You would like to see Mr. Ho Yin?" he inquired in impeccable English. "Then, please come with me."

I noticed a holster bulging from beneath his pajama top as we followed him a few blocks along the banyan-shaded waterfront promenade to the Bella Vista Hotel. The Bella Vista was a Mediterranean-style villa with a large marble patio overlooking the harbor. Cocktail hour dancers filled the patio, swaying to the muted playing of a Filipino band.

The little man motioned to a table, where we were to wait for Ho Yin. Despite his fluent English, our escort obviously wasn't strong on conversation. He then disappeared into the hotel.

We sat for an hour, sipping Madeira and watching the dancers. It was a beautiful evening. Junks, tied bow to stern, jammed the harbor, which appeared to reach all the way to China, just a mile away. Kerosene lanterns flickered from a thousand masts. Slowly, the moon rose over the whole scene, turning it into what could have been a travel poster for a tropical paradise. But Ho Yin never appeared.

Finally, our escort returned. There had been a mix-up, he explained. It was the Central Hotel where Ho Yin was waiting for us.

The Central was Macao's glittering gambling casino, packed every night with Portuguese prostitutes, high rollers from Hong Kong, and hundreds of Chinese playing fan tan, their favorite card game. Flanking the brightly lit casino entrance was a pair of Mozambique sentries. Half of Macao's security force was made up of these black soldiers from Portuguese Africa. They saluted us smartly, perhaps recognizing our escort as one of Ho Yin's minions.

The ground floor was lined with slot machines, or "coin-eating tigers" as they were called in Macao. As we entered, an angry woman practically yanked the iron arm off a machine. Apparently, it had eaten her last coin. At the same time, whistles, bells, and sirens were sounding farther down the line, signaling a jackpot.

Our pajama-clad guide pushed through the dense crowd, opening the way for us to a thickly carpeted back room furnished with overstuffed chairs. Again, he motioned to us to sit down. A white-coated waiter appeared, deposited two glasses and two bottles of orange soda on the polished blackwood table, and then vanished. "What kind of a cat-and-mouse game is this?" I wondered.

At last, the door opened a crack. A fat Chinese face half-hidden behind tinted glasses peered in. Then the door closed again. "He's sizing us up," I thought. "Can't decide if he really wants to meet us."

I was wrong. A few moments later, in strode Ho Yin, full of apologies for the mix-up in hotels and for making us wait. More important, he seemed amenable to our photographing his gold operation—or factory, as he called it.

The next day, in the steamy basement of the Tai Fong Bank among the furnaces and crucibles and sweating, half-naked workers, we received an education in how 400-troy-ounce, 99.6 percent-pure gold bricks were reduced in purity while smelting them into 99-percent-pure gold bars for the smugglers to transport to China. Actually, the smuggling syndicate trafficked in gold of all shapes and sizes, from whole bricks down to tiny gold beads that could be strapped to the legs of carrier pigeons. But the syndicate's biggest trade was in cigarette-size ten-tael (13.333-ounce) bars. Turning out almost a million dollars worth of these every day was the main business of Ho Yin's bank.

That was merely one part of the smuggling operation. We still had to find out from other sources how the gold was sneaked into China. So we hung around the harbor talking to the coolies who stowed the gold aboard the junks. For a wad of patacas (Macao currency), worth about ten dollars, they showed us the hiding places deep in the bilges, where even an honest Chinese customs inspector probably wouldn't think to look. The coolie stevedores also led us to two former U.S. Navy PT boats camouflaged to look like fishing launches. Outfitted with twin Packard engines, they could out run any Chinese customs vessel.

We were informed that the syndicate rarely used planes for the smuggling run to China. A few months earlier, two men who had boarded a flying boat bound for Hong Kong with several suitcases filled with gold bars in its baggage compartment tried to hijack the plane in mid-flight and succeeded in killing all twenty-two passengers, including themselves. The boat route was dangerous enough, often ending in gun battles with Chinese customs agents or with pirates infesting the South China Sea.

When the international edition of the magazine went on sale in Macao, P. J. Lobo took one look and ordered his flunkies to buy up all three thousand copies. He also declared Birns and me *persona non grata* in the Portuguese colony. Even though the magazine pictured him animatedly conducting his operetta *Cruel Separation* before a fawning crowd, he couldn't abide being called "Macao's real ruler who writes music to get his mind off gold."

Lobo's fury taught me two lessons I wouldn't forget. It demonstrated the impact an article could have on even the most remote flyspeck of a place. More importantly, it showed how thin-skinned local tyrants could be when light is shined directly on them. Lobo's gold syndicate (which he ran until he died in 1965) was an open secret in Macao. Yet, laying out the illicit smuggling operation in pictures and words for the rest of the world to see was another matter. Causing the biggest ruckus of all was the sequence of pictures showing in detail how the purity of the gold was reduced before it was recast into small, smuggling-size bars.

Life's picture story didn't show the gold entering Shanghai. The publicity surrounding our coverage may have forced Lobo's junks to land their precious cargoes in remote bays and coves along the lacy South China coast instead of sailing straight into Shanghai. Even if they did risk landing in Shanghai, members of the Macao syndicate could count on cooperation from the same corrupt customs agents I had encountered while patrolling the Huangpu River docks for CNRRA.

Before Ching-kuo resigned, he'd fought the Macao syndicate as best he could. He enlisted members of the Greater Shanghai Youth Service Corps to hang around the harbor and spy on the customs agents. He offered rewards to the sampan dwellers packed into Suzhou Creek to squeal on the smugglers. Nothing worked. Because of its growing instability, the city was simply too powerful a magnet for the yellow metal. It kept pouring in until Shanghai's whole economy became a raging black market pegged to gold.

Eventually, most of the smuggled gold spent to purchase food, clothing, and shelter found its way into the repositories of Shanghai's major banks. Ironically, it was the gold, whose flow into Shanghai Ching Kuo tried to halt, that his father, the generalissimo, was able to abscond with.

"Abscond" was certainly not the word Henry Luce would have chosen to describe the gold transfer to Taiwan ordered by his friend the Gimo. As *Time,* reflecting the proprietor's view, put it, "Chiang Kai-shek thoughtfully moved some $300 million of Nationalist gold to safer vaults in Formosa" (the Japanese name by which the island was then called). The magazine went on to explain: "If the Communists toppled the peace-seeking government of Acting President Li Zongren, the gold would serve as a nest egg for further resistance against the Reds."

The only trouble was Acting President Li wanted to get the "nest egg" back to curb inflation and pay the Nationalist troops in hard cash that were defending the Yangtze. He sent old Marshal Yan Xishan to Fenghua to plead with Chiang for return of the funds. According to *Time,* "the generalissimo listened politely, but refused to let go the gold."

By now, it was becoming clear to me that Luce was ready to let go of his fantasy that Mao Zedong's conquest of all China could still be curbed. Therefore, I was not surprised when in March 1949 an urgent cable came from *Life's* managing editor summoning me to New York for "an important meeting" with Luce. "The proprietor wants your eyewitness report on the current situation."

12

TALKS BEFORE THE ATTACK

The spring of 1949 marked a resting period for the Communist troops while they regrouped north of the Yangtze River. Acting President Li Zongren was also vying for time, hoping that he and his supporters could work out a peace compromise with Mao. This interlude in the fighting provided the perfect opportunity for me to fly to New York for my command performance with Henry Luce. Of course, he was more gracious than that about requesting my presence, cabling, "Please come at your own convenience."

However warmly the summons was phrased, I still was apprehensive. A feeling of uneasiness followed me all the way to the Time–Life Building in Rockefeller Center. Many of my correspondent friends in Shanghai assumed that Luce simply dictated the China policy of his magazines. That wasn't true. But the older China-hands, who were stationed in Chonquing during World War II, remembered the sign Teddy White posted on the shack that served as the *Time* bureau: ANY RESEMBLANCE TO WHAT IS WRITTEN HERE AND WHAT IS PRINTED IN *TIME* MAGAZINE, IS PURELY COINCIDENTAL. Even the American Consul General in Shanghai, John Moore Cabot, claimed, "Luce's idea of telling a story was to tell it the way it should have been, not the way it was." And, in China, that perception of Luce's distorted view of China, coupled with what was assumed to be his ironhanded control of editorial policy, never changed.

It was not an unreasonable assumption. After all, his birth and boyhood in China were well-known, and he often admitted to being "hopelessly sentimental" about the place. But the truth was that, while *Time,* his flagship publication, had been obliged to reflect his personal opinions, *Life* was free to print stories pretty much as we reported them.

"Sure, pictures don't lie," is how my friends at the Correspondents' Club in Shanghai dismissed the fact that *Life* didn't tamper with Birns' and my coverage. But these friends seemed to forget that our stories included sharply critical accounts of Chiang's military incompetence and Guomindang corruption—words that must have grated on Luce. Not that he brooked dissent about who controlled his magazines. He was the man in charge. But he applied different measuring sticks to what were then his only two weeklies.

Time certainly spoke for him and his company. And because it did, the magazine's editors were expected to rework the raw stuff that came in from the field. Not simply to insert Luce's sharply etched views of the world, but to forge an intellectual link between him and the magazine's readers. Once, to the dismay of everyone on the staff, he'd gone overboard and used that link to send a personal letter to all of *Time's* subscribers asking them to contribute to the United China Relief Fund.

Life was given a lot more latitude because of its emotional appeal. Its basic fare was the world as seen through the camera's viewfinder, and quite often that view didn't conform to Luce's. As a result, there were weeks when the two magazines presented divergent reports of China's civil war. But then, as Luce once told the staff, "It is the business of *Time* to make enemies, and *Life* to make friends." We reporters and photographers on *Life* appreciated our less confrontational role, even if our reporter friends in China didn't believe it.

When I started working for *Life* in Shanghai, bureau chief Bill Gray showed me a cable signed "HRL"—Henry Robinson Luce—that he received when he first arrived there. Bill thought it might be helpful for me to read it as I set forth on my new career in China.

"A brief statement of our journalistic and editorial policy toward Chinese affairs" is the way the cable began.

Luce then laid down certain "boundaries," as he called them, for what he considered *Time's* accurate, nonpartisan coverage. He made it clear that he accepted Chiang as a "loyal American ally," that *Time* would not support any "propagandistic efforts to overthrow him," and that "U.S. interests would be best served by an independent China, free of foreign domination of any sort."

Luce ended the cable saying, "This is not sent to you for your guidance in reporting the news. It is sent to you simply as sort of a first-aid kit to help you in the fierce partisan and propagandistic battle you may encounter in Asia." No mention was made of Teddy White, the man Bill had replaced. But the guidelines were clearly a warning not to take up White's anti-Chiang cudgel.

Afterward, when I was in Mukden or Taiyuan or some other besieged Chinese city, I sometimes wondered why Luce would disguise his guidelines as a "first-aid kit." Were they intended as bandages to bind any future wounds that Bill, or any other reporter working for the company, might incur during ideological clashes with the editor-in-chief? After all, not just Teddy White, but John Hersey, as well, fought hard with Luce over China—and quit. Both men were stars whom Luce hated to lose. Perhaps the first-aid kit was offered more as preventive medicine to keep Bill in a healthy frame of mind, and thus avoid the loss to the magazine of another talented reporter.

Those thoughts were flashing through my mind when Luce walked into the private dining room where we were about to have lunch. The large head with its receding hairline, the bushy eyebrows partially hiding piercing blue eyes, the corners of a mouth creased into a half smile, all matched the company portrait shot by his favorite *Life* photographer, Margaret Bourke-White.

I had only glimpsed the man once before, stepping quickly into an elevator. But the elevator operators in the Time–Life Building had orders to close the door right behind Luce, whisking him on a solo ride up to his thirty-third-floor office. That way he wasn't trapped into making small talk, which he hated.

Now, up close, he was shorter than I remembered. Perhaps my previous impression was thrown off by his predisposition for hiring very tall editors and publishers. In any case, here he was greeting me with a paternal pat on the shoulder, as if to confirm that I had done alright in my first year with *Life* and that he was glad to have me in his Time Inc. family.

It was my first time in one of the private, sixty-fourth-floor dining rooms atop what was then the RCA Building in Rockefeller Center. The view was magnificent. Straight ahead, standing like a sentinel over the city, the Empire State Building glistened in the midday sun. Beyond it, in shadow, the stunted buildings of Greenwich Village, where I had grown up, formed a dark valley that ended abruptly with another wall of sun-drenched skyscrapers rising from the financial district at the southern tip of Manhattan. I was suddenly reminded that it was in that dark valley that I had taken my first baby steps into journalism by publishing the *Bleecker Gardens Gazette,* that little mimeographed newspaper for the neighbors on my block. And here, fifteen years later, I was, part of a publishing behemoth with worldwide influence. And about to break bread with its founder.

Dissolving into the distant haze, the shimmering water of New York harbor spread out for miles, punctuated only by the tiny green Statue of Liberty. I was savoring this view, which was on the other side of the world from Shanghai in so many ways, when Luce motioned to the table for us to sit down.

To my surprise, Ed Thompson, then *Life*'s assistant managing editor (soon to be promoted to the magazine's top job) walked in. Ed's presence must have been a last-minute decision because only two places had been set at the table. A tuxedo-clad waiter quickly appeared with the cutlery and napkin for another setting. He also asked for drink orders, to which Ed eagerly responded by requesting a straight-up, double martini. Luce declined, and I followed his lead. Ed, I decided, had invited himself to lunch to jump in as my protector should I lock horns with Luce on China. The double martini would fortify him for such an emergency.

Luce seemed oblivious to the magnificent view. The private dining room might just as well have been a windowless cell. He got right down to discussing

Chiang Kai-shek and China, which obviously were the main items on the agenda. Luce had just finished escorting Madame Chiang around the U.S. on her most recent fundraising tour, and he didn't disguise his disappointment with the cool reception they got, especially Truman's contempt for Chiang and his wife.

On this trip, there had been no invitation to spend a night at the White House, where Madame Chiang had once brought her own satin sheets. Or to speak to Congress, which only recently had given Chiang another $1 billion. Truman did not simply turn down the Madame's appeal for more money, he issued a testy statement to the press reminding the world that American aid to China already exceeded $3.8 billion. "They're a bunch of thieves, every damn one of them," Truman remarked later, referring to the Nationalist leaders. "They stole $750 million of the billions we sent to Chiang."

As the lunch progressed, I thought the editor-in-chief showed himself to be a man of contradictions, just as John Hersey once described him.

> *He was shy, yet candid. He was very opinionated, but he was also consumed with curiosity. At one moment he sounded cold and controlled, the next moment he was full of boyish enthusiasm. He was bright, all right. But as his mind darted and jumped, several ideas seemed to be trying to escape from his mouth at once, causing a slight stammer.*

I was amazed, however, to hear that he no longer held any illusions about saving Chiang's crumbling regime. Oh yes, he had expected Mao's "Godless revolution" to fail. Right up until the Nationalists lost Manchuria, he admitted he still retained hope that Chiang would prevail. He even complimented me on my eyewitness description in *Life* of the Mukden debacle, claiming it helped to convince him of Chiang's ultimate defeat. He confessed that after Mukden's fall he had put pressure on Truman to send more military and economic aid. He'd also searched, he said, for splits within the Guomindang Party—a development that I had reported on in *Life*—that might have spawned a more popular movement in China to resist the fast-moving Red tide. But, unfortunately, he added, none appeared.

"Now," lamented Luce, "it's too late for outside aid or for internal political repairs." Even Ed Thompson was taken aback by Luce's acceptance of Chiang Kai-shek's hopeless situation and the certainty of his defeat.

But there was nothing defeatist about Luce. He struck me as being too bright and upbeat for that. After hearing my dismal appraisal of the war, and delivering his own, he dwelled on happier days, when he was a "mishkid," as the sons and daughters of American missionaries in China were called. He described the avid fundraising his father had done for Yenching University. He mentioned that he even once thought of becoming a businessman in China because of "the big economic opportunities in a country where everybody had their nose to the grindstone." But, after starting *Time*, his determination to participate in China's economic development, he said, "was confined to supporting Chiang's modernization efforts."

Suddenly ending this philosophic soliloquy, Luce started firing questions at me. "How long will it take Mao's troops to regroup before sweeping on south?" "How long can Nanjing and Shanghai hold out?" "Will a wave of panic paralyze those two cities before the Communists march in?" "When do you expect Chiang, who is still living in supposed retirement in Fenghua, to flee to Formosa?"

As he continued to pepper me with questions about the Nationalists' impending collapse, I noticed how he cocked his head slightly to the left, carefully weighing each answer. He was a good listener. I wondered whether William Randolph Hearst, or Colonel Robert McCormick, or any of the other press lords with such immense power and influence, would have been so receptive to the ideas of a lowly reporter. That, I decided, was one of Luce's most attractive qualities.

After I answered his last query, he lapsed into descriptions of his most recent visits to China. He'd met Mao in Chongqing in 1945, he said, but confessed to being appalled by the Communist leader's "sloppy dress and peasant-like look." At the same time, he said, he'd enjoyed "a wonderfully relaxed and frank chat" with Zhou Enlai, even though Zhou complained that *Time* hadn't been very nice to him recently.

I described to Luce Zhou Enlai's surprise visit to the UNRRA compound in Kaifeng when I was working there and how tough he'd been in insisting that the Communists get their share of the relief supplies. I also described how witty and urbane he proved to be during the dinner conversation. Luce said he'd noticed that same Jekyll and Hyde trait in Zhou.

The fact that that Zhou and Mao were Communists clearly hadn't lessened Luce's eagerness to meet them. As a publisher, he obviously enjoyed mingling with the power-elite whose lives his magazines chronicled. In the original prospectus for *Life*, before the magazine's birth when it was tentatively still being called *Show-Book of the World*, Luce had defined its purpose this way: "To see life; to see the world; to eyewitness great events; to watch the faces of the poor and the gestures of the proud." Clearly, he was a spirited enough reporter to enjoy doing all of those things himself.

Luce described how, on that same trip to China, he had also visited Qingdao, where as a boy he and his family had spent many happy vacations. "It's the most beautiful place on earth," he recalled, relating how the mountains drop straight down to the Yellow Sea. He explained that Kaiser Wilhelm II, after grabbing Qingdao for Germany in 1898, referred to it as "the fairest jewel in his crown." "All I wanted to do on that return visit was swim on the beaches of the bay as I did when I was a boy," Luce added.

Some years later, after Mao was firmly in control of China, Luce was telling a group of us about that same visit to Qingdao. Again, he mentioned going swimming and how he was accompanied by General Lemuel Shepherd, whom he described as "the finest swimmer in the United States Marine Corps." "If American affairs had been entrusted to General Shepherd and me, China would not now be Communist," said Luce.

Reminiscing some more for Ed Thompson and me, Luce told us about another visit to China in 1946. He was there, he said, for the generalissimo's birthday, and recalled going on a "beautiful and memorable outing" arranged by Madame Chiang.

"We traveled for about two hours on a private train," said Luce, "to a large lake where we boarded a houseboat and were served a delicious lunch. After lunch we came upon an island with an ancient temple." There were steamer chairs in front of the temple, Luce said, and described how he and the generalissimo both "stretched out for a long nap in the warm November sunshine." From Luce's description, I recognized it as the unusual "lake within the lake" in Hangzhou, a resort town about one hundred miles southwest of Shanghai. It was a place where we correspondents occasionally went for a little R and R.

Luce said that during the trip he also spent several evenings in Nanjing dining with American Ambassador John Leighton Stuart, whom he referred to as "an old missionary friend of my father's."

"I was briefed extensively," Luce explained, "by both the ambassador and by General Marshall, who was still trying to mediate peace between the Nationalists and the Communists." But, according to Luce, Stuart had come to the opposite conclusion about China from Marshall. He believed the only solution was American support of Chiang, including the use of American troops if necessary.

"So we had an ironic situation," recalled Luce. "The man of God favoring military action, and the soldier unwilling to use the sword." In the years that followed, I heard Luce repeat that wonderful line several times.

It was almost three o'clock when he interrupted his reminiscences with the reminder, "Time to get back to work."

Before we broke up, he confided that just a few months ago, while Birns and I were with General Li Mi covering the million-man battle for Xuzhou, he had fired off an angry letter to Republican Senator Arthur Vandenburg about the U.S. government's shabby treatment of the generalissimo. Luce didn't say much else about the contents of the letter. But, after he died, I read that Luce had complained bitterly to Vandenburg about being perceived as "a guy peddling America's vital interest in China as if it were some sort of bottled chop suey that I was trying to sneak through the Pure Food Laws"—another wonderfully funny line from this serious editor-in-chief not known for his wit.

As we headed for the elevator, Luce mentioned that he'd also written a personal letter to Chiang Kai-shek. "It was," he said, "my final plea for the generalissimo to come out of retirement to defend the Yangtze, and at the same time to broaden his government so that it represented all the non-Communist elements in China." He ended the letter by recommending that the generalissimo move the capital from besieged Nanjing to the temporary safety of Guangzhou.

"And that reminds me," said the editor-in-chief as we shook hands, "when and where should we move the Shanghai bureau?"

"Hong Kong," I answered. "From there we'll be able to keep a close watch on China. And it's the biggest transportation hub in Southeast Asia."

I could see disappointment spread across Luce's face. The idea of his magazines having to abandon the country of his birth was clearly painful.

"Could we stay in Shanghai under the Communists?" he asked, then answered the question himself. "No, Time Inc. couldn't do that."

That memorable lunch with Luce quickly faded into a distant dream, or so it seemed, as I flew back to China and plunged once again into covering the war, or more precisely, the remote possibility of a peaceful settlement. But my correspondent friends in Shanghai and Nanjing were now talking about the "black hand" of Chiang as the biggest obstacle to peace. A liberal Shanghai newsletter, the *Far Eastern Bulletin,* even dared to go public with the same thought. "His ubiquitous hand in the shadow," it stated, "has never ceased to direct the whole political-military scene south of the Yangtze." The publication went on to complain that "from his control tower in Fenghua, Chiang is keeping each of the Guomindang Party factions so weak that the door is wide open for his comeback." Ambassador Stuart made a similar observation in a report to the State Department. "The generalissimo is interfering in military affairs," he wrote, "thus hampering rather than helping the Yangtze defense."

Reports like those continued to undermine Vice President Li Zongren's authority. Li still believed that if he could get a three-month respite from the Communists, the Nationalists might be able to reorganize and keep Mao's forces from crossing the Yangtze. Mao, he reckoned, also understood the cost of taking the south by force, and would therefore prefer a peaceful settlement.

To explore the peace possibilities, Li sent a group of prominent Shanghai businessmen to meet with the Communists in the northern town of Xibaipo. The group held brief preliminary meetings with Mao and Zhou Enlai. Two weeks later, Li sent a bigger group to Xibaipo with a mandate to work out a framework for negotiations. Not surprisingly, Zhou gave Li's representatives a good working over, finally getting them to agree to the Communists' stringent terms. When the peace delegates reported back to Li Zongren, he was horrified that they hadn't been able to wring a few concessions from the Communists.

After receiving intelligence reports of Li's peace efforts, Chiang became more agitated than ever. He suspected that Li and his deputies were preparing to defect. Referring now to his "temporary resignation," the generalissimo once again asserted control over the Nationalist armies defending the lower reaches of the Yangtze, including Shanghai. At the same time, he continued to build Taiwan into a military stronghold.

For Mao, the big question was where and how to cross the Yangtze under fire. He assumed that the Nationalist Army, Navy, and Air Force, with possible support from the U.S. Navy, would try to repel the crossing. In Beijing, secret negotiations had been going on with defectors from the Nationalist Navy to grant the Communists free passage. Even so, Mao realized the crossing would be dangerous.

In late March, he appointed a committee, headed by Zhou Enlai and General Lin Biao, to negotiate with another group of Li Zongren's representatives, this one led by the hard-headed former Nationalist commander in Xinjiang Province, General Zhang Zhizhong. Once again, the Communists shocked Li's emissaries by demanding what amounted to full surrender. The Nationalists were given a two-week deadline to accept. Faced with that ultimatum, Li then made one last desperate attempt to get the U.S. and the other Western powers to save his regime. The request was flatly rejected. In the words of Ambassador Stuart, "Li was obviously disheartened, chilled by our reserved, somewhat formal response."

In early April, still serving as acting president, Li telegraphed a final plea for mercy to Mao. "To convert hostilities into peace and to save the people," he wired the Communist leader, "I will accept without evasion the severest punishment, even to the extent of being boiled in oil, or having my physical self dismembered into many parts as a so-called war criminal."

No victor in China's millennial history ever received a more complete admission of defeat than this telegram. "Your message has been received," Mao wired back. "Our party is willing to adopt lenient terms."

For another week, the Nationalists and Communists bargained and bickered over what "lenient" meant. The Nationalists petitioned for an "equal and honorable" peace. The Communists shouted back, "That's mad and erroneous. There is only one way to peace, and that is by complete surrender." Mao finally drafted an ultimatum and sent it south to Nanjing by messenger. "Within four days," he demanded, "all Nationalist troops must be put under Communist command."

Clearly, Mao's heart was with his soldiers, not in negotiations. When Li Zongren failed to hand over his armies, Mao followed his own famous axiom: "Power flows from the barrel of a gun." On April 20, he ordered his forces to "advance boldly and resolutely to thoroughly, cleanly, and completely annihilate all those who dare to resist."

On April 21, seven hours before the ultimatum's deadline, Mao's shock troops jammed onto river craft and struck across the Yangtze in a vast envelopment operation. Three advance groups from the two-million-man Communist army made the initial assault. The first group, from Chen Yi's Third Field Army, crossed the river half way between Nanjing and Shanghai. The second group, from Lin Biao's Fourth Field Army, aimed directly at Nanjing, crossing the river both east and west of the Nationalist capital. The third group, from Liu Bocheng's Second Field Army, crossed the river southwest of Nanjing, splitting off the coastal area from the interior.

"The river rang with silvery notes of bugles and martial music," exulted the Communist radio. "Boats by the thousands shuttled between the northern and southern banks, as one thousand guns belched fire and smoke, lighting the Yangtze waters in a lurid glare."

The Nationalists' Twenty-sixth Army, which had been ordered by Acting President Li to defend the city, never arrived. Local defenses quickly crumbled for lack of coordination and for failure of the commanders to take orders from anyone but the generalissimo, who was still officially retired in Fenghua. Chiang's generals knew that he wanted them to concentrate on the defense of Shanghai and the coastal provinces rather than trying to slow the assault on Nanjing. Making the attack even more one sided, the entire Nationalist river navy defected to the Communists.

Life had sent photographer Carl Mydans from Tokyo to help me cover the hurried evacuation of the Nationalist capital. Called "Stump" because of his short, stocky build, Carl was one of the magazine's original photographers. He and his reporter wife, Shelley, had been captured by the Japanese in the Philippines at the start of World War II and were held prisoners in Manila and in Shanghai before being repatriated on the Swedish liner *Gripsholm.*

I had never met Carl, but by one of those funny coincidences, our paths almost crossed. Three years after the Japanese released him, *Life* sent Carl back to Manila to photograph the freeing of his former fellow prisoners. Shortly after that, the army assigned me to the landing craft company in Manila's port. One day, the public relations chief for the Armed Forces of the Western Pacific approached me breathlessly. "Could you zip out to one of the Liberty ships anchored in the bay and commandeer a turkey?" he asked. "It's for the famous *Life* photographer Carl Mydans." That was as close as I'd ever come to encountering Carl.

Now, as we watched the long lines of frightened Nationalist soldiers fleeing Nanjing ahead of the Communists, Carl said it reminded him of the day he was photographing the crowds of panicked American civilians trying to escape from Manila ahead of the Japanese. "That's when I was captured. But

I'll never surrender again!" he exclaimed. "Next time I'll run and risk getting shot in the back."

Most of the American wives and children had already left Nanjing, ferried down the river on a U.S. Navy landing craft. So had General Barr's Military Advisory Group, sent to China by President Truman to teach the Nationalists modern warfare. Only six U.S. Marines remained to guard the embassy.

We discovered that Barr and his officers had left so hurriedly they couldn't decide what to take and what to leave. Of course, all remaining documents were burned—"with the odor of red tape," I noted cynically. Destroyed also, but for reasons that didn't make sense, were some 14,000 Armed Forces Radio transcriptions. They had been used to bombard Nanjing with just about every kind of entertainment, from Bob Hope to Spike Jones. "Those tapes would have confused the shit out of the Commies," commented the sergeant, who had been ordered to destroy them. But he declared proudly that the supreme achievement of the whole hurried American evacuation was his rescue of some 30,000 cases of beer, barged down the river to Shanghai.

Chinese civilians left just about all of their possessions behind. Cursing, bribing, and fighting, they surged aboard any train or boat that would carry them away from the Nationalist capital. I had never witnessed such chaos, not even in Mukden or Taiyuan.

Finally, Nanjing lay quiet. Streetlights still flickered wanly until the 11:00 P.M. curfew, then blinked out. After that, the streets were deserted except for rifle-toting municipal gendarmes wearing shabby black uniforms and yellow armbands.

Daylight did nothing to lift the funereal mood of the city. At Sun Yat-sen Circle, in midtown, the loudspeaker that used to blare out Strauss waltzes was silent. The throngs of shouting, arm-waving money changers had dwindled to a few individuals. The price of their clinking stacks of silver dollars kept on climbing dizzily. There was no shortage of these coins because the Nationalist soldiers were now being paid in silver to keep them from defecting.

At the old Ming Palace Airport inside the city wall, salvage crews belonging to the Da Hwa Hardware Company were busy cutting up the last aluminum wings and fuselages of wrecked Chinese Air Force planes. Melted down in furnaces right on the field, the molten aluminum was then poured into ingots to be used for making kitchen utensils. "Instead of turning swords into plowshares," I jotted in my notebook, "the Chinese are converting American war surplus planes into pots and pans. Wouldn't that piss off our taxpayers!"

It was 3:30 in the morning on April 22, 1949, when the Communists began their attack on the city. Li Zongren was in Hangzhou trying to convince Chiang Kai-shek to join him in a concerted plan of resistance. With promises of cooperation from the generalissimo, Li flew back to the capital just as it was being cut off by the Communists. He met with his advisors that night. "We will fight to the bitter end," they promised. "Nanjing will hold out for six months." But at dawn, Li along with Premier Ho Yinching and Nanjing's garrison commander, sped to the airport. Soldiers put them aboard waiting planes, hastily jumped in after them, and slammed the doors.

Most of the gendarmes changed quickly into civilian clothes. The rest disappeared as a wave of looting swept the city. At Acting President Li's abandoned gray brick home, I watched a mob swarm up the long, tree-lined driveway. A boy shoved a porcelain sink through a smashed door to his friends outside. "The sooner they clean out the place, the better," explained Li's housekeeper, who helped the looters remove scrolls and furniture.

The flowerbeds in Mayor Teng Chieh's gardens were littered with broken glass and pieces of plaster. There, I watched a man wrestle with a steam radiator, trying to lift it onto his shoulder. "I didn't like the mayor anyway," he said. Later I learned that the mayor had tried to escape in his car loaded with 300 million gold yuan, only to be beaten up by his chauffeur and bodyguard before being captured by the Communists.

At a food shop, coolies shoved their way through the crowd to confiscate the few remaining sacks of flour. A man who was empty-handed jumped onto the back of a little fellow lugging a sack away. They rolled together into the gutter. When Mydans started to take their picture, a young Chinese woman cried out in English, "No, no, you must not. This is a disgrace."

Before dawn the next day, 20,000 troops of Chen Yi's Third Field Army marched into the capital. Country boys from Shandong stared in wonder at Nanjing's modern government buildings while university students gathered to sing patriotic songs of welcome. The troops were armed with an assortment of weapons, including Japanese rifles, but mostly with captured American sub-machine guns. Some carried baskets of vegetables dangling from shoulder poles.

The foreign community, surprisingly, was almost ignored. However, a dozen People's Liberation Army soldiers sightseeing around the city forced the night watchmen at the American embassy to open the iron gates. Three soldiers then barged into Ambassador Stuart's second-floor bedroom. "Who are you?" shouted the seventy-two-year-old envoy. "What do you want?" After telling him that "all the things in this house will eventually belong to the people," they left.

Even the Communist generals couldn't resist playing around in the presidential palace. Deng Xiaoping would recount later how he and General Chen Yi took turns sitting in the generalissimo's chair.

13

SHOOTING "THE LAST DAYS OF SHANGHAI"

For Shanghai's foreign community, the attack on Nanjing was just one more step in the Communists' march south—no more frightning than the siege of Mukden, Beijing, or Taiyuan. Nor did it come as any surprise. After prolonged peace talks and several surrender ultimatums, everybody expected it. Besides, Shanghai—*their* city, not the Nationalist capital—was the beating heart of China.

That ostrich-like attitude amazed me. Except for soaring inflation and spasmodic gold rushes—accepted as mere inconveniences—life in Shanghai hadn't changed dramatically. But how could thousands of American, British, and French businessmen and their wives and children be so unconcerned? They acted as if the fighting was taking place in another part of the world. The Cold War and Berlin blockade were getting a bigger play in Shanghai's four English-language dailies. The city's neon glow, and the nightlife associated with it, hadn't dimmed. Caviar and vodka flowed freely as ever at Kafka's, the best Russian restaurant in town. And you could still party the hours away at Ciros, the Metropole, and Lido despite a loosely enforced curfew, which the Park Hotel circumvented by advertising "dinner dancing under the moon" starting at 6:00 P.M.

At home, husbands and wives were reluctant to discuss what one of them described to me as "this bothersome war." But then, like unwilling spectators of a still-distant clash over which they had no control, their own safety had yet to be jeopardized. And, for that matter, neither had their luxurious lifestyle, made possible by a full retinue of servants at home, and by those indispensable "compradors" (Chinese fixers) who smoothed out problems at the office. Some foreigners speculated that business might actually improve under the Communists.

Jack Cabot, the American Consul General, said, "At first I had to shout at all our women and children trying to persuade them to leave. Then I spent months trying to stop them from coming back." He claimed the State Department was just as blasé. "I sent Washington a list of evacuation priorities, but never got a reply." British Consul General Robert Urquhart, on the other hand, found little to worry about. At a closed meeting held at the Columbia Country Club on Bubbling Well Road, he assured British businessmen that all they had to do was "be patient and prepare for the resumption of full trading activities."

Then, without warning, a series of violent incidents on the Yangtze River sent shockwaves through Shanghai. Carl Mydans and I were still in Nanjing covering the Nationalist evacuation, unaware of the panic suddenly gripping Shanghai or of the amount of bloodshed on the river. It was a week before I could interview one of the survivors for a blow-by-blow account of what happened.

Steaming slowly upriver on April 20, the Royal Navy sloop *Amethyst* and its 183-man crew was headed for Nanjing with a load of supplies for British subjects caught in the teetering capital. A Union Jack was painted on each side of her gray steel hull as she plowed the silted waters. Most of the crew was still at breakfast when two Communist artillery shells landed twenty yards from the ship, sending up great geysers of water. Everyone aboard assumed the Communists were firing at the Nationalist troops defending the south bank and that a few shells had fallen short of their mark. The firing soon stopped, and the *Amethyst* proceeded on course.

Half an hour later, as she negotiated a sharp bend in the river, two shells smashed into the *Amethyst*'s bridge and wheelhouse. Her rudder controls jammed, and the wounded sloop twisted helplessly in the current until she ran aground on the mud flats off Rose Island. Although her forward guns were pointed in the wrong direction, her stern guns began shelling the Communist positions. The Communist shore batteries cut loose again. Within minutes, the captain of the *Amethyst* was mortally wounded, and many of the members of the crew, including the ship's doctor and pharmacist's mate, were dead.

Most of the survivors, I was told, were issued rifles and ordered to abandon ship, leaving just a skeleton crew aboard. Every lifeboat but one had been smashed, so only the wounded and those who couldn't swim were put in it. The others jumped overboard and swam to the island. Nationalist troops, dug in on the south bank, finally realized it was a British ship that had been attacked and sent sampans across the narrow channel to the island to rescue the stranded sailors.

When news of the river battle flashed through Nanjing, the first question British residents asked was, "Are we at war?" Old Brits in the city, harking back to their glory days of gunboat diplomacy, expected instant retaliation by their government. That, I assumed, would also have been the reaction of any longtime American residents recalling the Japanese bombing of the U.S. gunboat *Panay*, when it was seeking to evacuate embassy personnel from Nanjing in 1937.

Mao, too, according to his biographers, wondered if the British would retaliate. At the moment of the attack, he was in Beijing awaiting word on the foreign community's reaction to his assault on Nanjing. He expected most of the foreign embassies would stay put. Stalin had even recommended to him that, after Nanjing fell, the Communists should conduct "businesslike relations" with the capitalist powers there.

But, after the attack on the *Amethyst*, Mao was no longer sure if that would be possible. However, the mere presence of a British gunboat on the Yangtze was too much a symbol of what he considered the old China to be ignored, especially at the precise moment his People's Liberation Army was poised to make its hazardous river crossing. In fact, he had instructed his field commanders to "brook no foreign interference with the taking of Nanjing." That explained why his troops had opened fire on the *Amethyst.* They figured the British warship had come to block their crossing of the Yangtze.

Of course, Mao's orders were not known at the time. Carl and I couldn't understand what could have prompted a British warship to get caught in a firefight with the Communists. Our first instinct was to head downriver for Rose Island, expecting the RAF might be called in to bomb the Communist positions. Then we discovered we'd have to cross Communist lines to get there, and that would have been foolhardy with more than a million of Mao's troops infiltrating the area.

If we'd realized that the battle to save the British sloop was just beginning, Carl and I might have risked it. Or if we'd known the British frigate *Consort* was about to speed downriver from Nanjing to try to rescue the *Amethyst,* we'd have tried to talk our way on board. The situation was so confusing we finally opted to remain in Nanjing until the last moments before the Communists entered the city.

As we learned later, the *Consort* took off immediately after receiving the *Amethyst's* SOS to lend whatever assistance she could. When Mao heard that the British frigate, as well as the 10,000-ton cruiser *London,* had set sail for Rose Island, he telegraphed his generals that the two British warships "should *not* be attacked unless they interfere with our military operations." But Mao's message arrived too late. When the *Consort* reached Rose Island that afternoon, the Communist batteries, which were still raking the *Amethyst* with fire, turned their guns on the frigate, killing eight members of her crew and wounding thirty. After flashing a message of encouragement to the skeleton crew left on the *Amethyst,* the crippled *Consort* limped away. By the time the firing finally stopped, the *Amethyst* had been hit by fifty-three shells. Twenty-three members of her crew were dead or dying, and thirty-one others were wounded.

The *London* never got within sight of the *Amethyst.* Built to fight in open water, the heavily armed cruiser proved even more helpless in the Yangtze than the two smaller ships. The Communists riddled her vulnerable super-structure, and before she got back to Shanghai, shells tore some twenty-five holes in her hull. One shell exploded in an ammunition locker, killing fifteen crewmembers and wounding twenty others. Like the *Consort,* the *London* had to turn back, but not before radioing the *Amethyst* with typical British understatement, "Sorry, we cannot help you today."

The first contingent from the *Amethyst*—those who had swum ashore—reached Shanghai by train on the afternoon of April 21, and were transported by bus to the British Consulate. Mrs. Urquhart, wife of the consul general, had telephoned a number of the British wives with spare rooms in their homes to take in one or two of the survivors for the night. As Noel Barber reported in his book *The Fall of Shanghai,* "No one knew exactly what time the train would arrive, so the ladies gathered in the consulate early and played bridge until the fifty-three men arrived from the station around five o'clock, dirty, ragged, and unshaven, many barefooted, all looking utterly dejected."

Hearing about the attack on the *London,* Carl and I rushed back to Shanghai in time to see the battered cruiser limp into port. I jotted in my notebook, "The crowds of stunned British and American spectators looked as shell-shocked as the severely wounded sailors being carried ashore." No less stunned, I also noted, were "Shanghai's city officials, who realized that the Communists had done something no Chinese army ever dared do before—blow the warships of a Western power out of one of its rivers."

Mao, of course, as we eventually learned from Communist accounts, was elated. He told his generals, "The incidents with the British warships have shaken the world, and become the headlines of all the main newspapers in Britain and America." He also thought he detected a change in the attitude of the imperialist powers. "The Americans are asking people to pass messages to us for the establishment of diplomatic relations," he wrote (although that didn't happen until three decades later). "The British are trying hard to engage in business with us."

The British government's timid reaction surprised its subjects more than the incident itself. For more than a century, the Royal Navy had enjoyed complete supremacy in China, attacking here and there with little provocation. In the so-called Arrow War of 1856 it hit Tianjin simply because Chinese officials took it upon themselves to search a coastal steamer (the *Arrow*) flying the Union Jack. Now, all that British Consul General Urquhart would say is, "We think we have the situation under control." But, as the *New York Times* reported, "With the likelihood increasing that South China, too, will be overrun by the Communist armies, the British are not willing to involve themselves in a dispute with the Communist leaders that might end in the complete loss of British property." It was a point echoed by British taipans in Shanghai, who, Noel Barber reported, could be heard saying things like, "My dear fellow, we've got millions tied up in China, to say nothing of the thousands of our countrymen who earn good money here."

The U.S. State Department was still deeply divided on how to deal with the Chinese Communist leader and was unwilling to break with the generalissimo, a move Mao insisted on for the establishment of diplomatic relations. The British, despite the attack on their ships, were nevertheless ready to switch allegiance and recognize the Communists as soon as Shanghai fell.

Shanghai was too boisterous, too unruly, too much of a throbbing metropolis to die the quick death of Nanjing. Historically, it had always been a hive of colliding ideas, including the birthplace of China's Communist Party. Old residents remembered that the party's plenary session in 1921 had been held there. And that this young man Mao, who had been drifting around town discussing the *Communist Manifesto* and other Marxist texts that had just been translated into Chinese, represented his home province of Hunan at the meeting. Still, nobody in Shanghai ever dreamed that twenty-eight years later a victorious Mao would stand ready to conquer their city.

As the warm May evenings brought big crowds back to the riverfront park behind the Bund, people now tried hard to hide their fear. Shopkeepers pretended it was business as usual even though inflation had soared into the stratosphere. I saw a rickshaw boy dive headlong for a cigarette butt but ignore a 100 GY note lying in the street. Still, the virtually worthless currency didn't stop the buying and selling that was the soul of Shanghai. Deals continued in U.S. dollars, gold bars, or by barter. As usual, the carefully cen-sored Nationalist newspapers also did their best to put the public at ease. The *Chung Yang Jih-pao,* in describing the fall of Nanjing, commented that "a strategic withdrawal must not be confused with a military defeat."

My own reporting of the false calm pervading Shanghai didn't slake the ap-petite of *Life's* desk-bound editors in New York for more war coverage. They seemed to be salivating for what they called "a poignant photographic essay on the dying city," and kept badgering me for a timetable of Shanghai's demise.

"For planning purposes need best guess when city will fall," queried as-signment editor Bill Churchill. "State Department warns Shanghai garrison planning last-ditch defense. Do you expect street-by-street fight, or quick surrender?"

Only the "double-domers," as we China correspondents called the crys-tal ball-gazing political analysts in the Washington press corps, could answer questions like that. And I suggested to the editors, perhaps a bit rudely, that they contact one of them. But my curt message didn't stop the barrage of re-quests from New York. "Whatever happens, want stark, gutsy 'Last Days of Shanghai' essay," wired Wilson Hicks, the picture editor. "Need stirring eye-witness account," chimed in foreign editor Filmore Calhoun with yet an-other cabled request.

Nobody in our editorial offices in New York knew what was going to happen. Yet they all knew precisely what kind of pictures and words they wanted to appear under the headline "The Last Days of Shanghai," on the assumption that there would be no life left to speak of once the Communists took over.

The problem for photographer Jack Birns and me was that Shanghai didn't look like it was living out its "last days." The sights and sounds hadn't changed much with the approach of the Communists. Dice still rattled atop the mahogany bar of the American Club. Only now those noontime dice players called themselves the "Die-hards." The Brits, likewise, continued their beloved afternoon lawn bowl games, fueled by the usual number of pink gins—but with one alteration. Rolls of concertina barbed wire enclosed their manicured greensward to keep out potential rioters. And the ping of tennis balls could still be heard all day long at the Le Cercle Sportif Française. Residents of the French Concession were unperturbed. As far as they were concerned, Shanghai would remain the "Paris of the East" even under the Communists, just as those who knew Shanghai as the "Whore of Asia" expected it would continue living up to that name, too. Business had slowed in the honky-tonks of Hongkew. But a sailor on the prowl could still find hookers aplenty perched on the bar stools at Duke Lear's, or Bob Brown's Diamond Bar, or the Tango, or Rainbow—though not at Frank Yenalevicz's New Ritz Bar in Blood Alley. "Yen" never did allow "hostesses" in his place, and he still didn't. "You wanna buy this joint?" he asked me facetiously. "Some dope offered me forty thousand last year. I couldn't give it away today."

For the fifty foreign correspondents living in Broadway Mansions, life there was little changed. The lower floors had already been vacated by the departing American military personnel, so we had the whole building to ourselves. The only sign of an impending battle was the shouted commands of troops holding close-order drills on the garage roof directly below my fifteenth-floor bedroom window.

"You stay Shanghai?" my room boy inquired hopefully. "Stay Shanghai as long as I can," I replied. But he saw through my feigned optimism and shook his head.

My morning walk to the Time–Life office kept to its old routine. Crossing the Garden Bridge spanning the Suzhou Creek, I paused, as usual, to watch the "push boys" chase the torrent of pedicabs, offering a helping shove going up the steep incline, then hanging on going down the other side of the bridge until the rider produced a tip. Although now, with food prices soaring, a pedicab going over the bridge loaded with sacks of rice instead of a passenger risked being pounced on by ruffians armed with ice picks. Quickly puncturing a bag or two, they would catch handfuls—or, more often, hatfuls—of rice pouring out of the ruptured bags before the pedaler realized he was under attack.

The wide waterfront promenade along the Bund continued to pulsate with those practicing the ancient art of *tai chi chuan*. A pair of blind beggars who were there every morning staring out of empty eye sockets greeted me, as always, with outstretched palms. They were able to tell the sound of my footsteps from all the rest, and being on my daily payroll, so to speak, showed no sign of giving up their profitable positions.

Unlike in Nanjing, the big companies in Shanghai belonged to foreigners. The Brits still ran the waterworks, wharves, shipping, banks, and trolley cars, while the power plants, telephone, and gas companies were owned and operated by Yanks. Most of the Old China-hand managers had weathered wars and uprisings before, and had no plans to leave. Their only immediate problem was protecting their posh homes in Honqiao. That fashionable western suburb had been picked by the Shanghai garrison for its last stand against the Communists. And Nationalist General Tang Enbo, appointed by the generalissimo to defend the city, had vowed, "Shanghai will be China's Stalingrad." He boasted that he would make the inner city impenetrable by the construction of a wooden stockade, though most people suspected it was simply a plan to enrich a timber merchant friend.

When Birns began photographing the army's defense preparations in Honqiao, a colonel tried to wrest the camera away. *"Buhao! Buhao!"* ("very bad, very bad"), he shouted, knowing that every foreigner recognized those two Chinese words. But he quickly disappeared, and Birns resumed his picture-taking.

Here, at least, was some photographable action for our "Last Days of Shanghai" essay. We found one squad of soldiers ripping up the headstones from the Hongqiao cemetery to form protective shields around their machine gun positions. Another squad was dynamiting trees, leveling hedges, and burning down houses to open an unobstructed field of fire. Even the Honqiao Golf Club was being torn down, although we noticed that its ceramic roof tiles had been carefully removed and set aside for future use.

The razing and burning was being carried out in almost a carnival spirit. "Those soldiers are having a wonderful time destroying what their foreign masters spent decades building," observed Randall Gould, the acerbic American editor of the *Shanghai Evening Post and Mercury.*

We moved on to the lavish twenty-acre Jardine, Matheson and Company estate. The British firm's imposing managing director, John Keswick, and his wife Clare, had just had their breakfast interrupted by a fresh-faced young officer. Behind the officer we saw several soldiers holding baskets of wood shavings. Obviously, they had come to burn down the Keswick house.

"Young man, I was living in this house before you were born," roared Sir John. "This is our home and we intend to stay here."

Keswick was the biggest taipan in town. His company owned the EWO textile mill, Holt's Wharf, the Shanghai-Honkew Wharf, and numerous other buildings and enterprises. The giant conglomerate had grown out of a small opium trading company founded in 1832 by Keswick's great-great uncle, Dr. William Jardine. A shrewd Scotsman, Jardine had written, "If the opium trade is ever legalized, our business will cease to be profitable." But family continuity and tenacity, not opium, resulted in the firm's survival and prosperity.

"Three times," bellowed Sir John, "I was forced to evacuate Shanghai, and I'm not going to let you people or the Communists drive me out again."

The young officer stared at the glowering figure, not knowing how to respond. On a map that showed all the houses to be demolished, he slowly drew a circle around the Keswicks' estate, indicating that this one spot could be spared, at least for the moment.

As we were leaving, Sir John handed us a copy of a book by him titled *What I Know About China.* "I had this published in England," he said. "It's been quite popular. This is the third edition." It was an unusual book, all right. Beautifully bound, it consisted of one hundred blank pages, a stunning admission from an Old China-hand with Keswick's experience.

Several families besides the Keswicks were holding out in Hongqiao. Nearby, at an estate called The Limit because it was the last house on the city's southwest boundary, *Time* correspondent Bob Doyle looked in on Mrs. Gladys Hawkings. By the time he arrived, soldiers had already pulled down fences on neighboring properties, dug trenches through the gardens, and started chopping down trees. When one group of soldiers started chopping down Mrs. Hawkings's trees, she flew out of the house and started scolding them in Chinese. The soldiers were overwhelmed by her bearing and perfect Chinese. Obediently, they put away their axes.

Mrs. Hawkings then took Doyle into the pantry, where she and her husband planned to hole up if fighting erupted around their house. "The bathroom is overhead," she explained, "and that has a thick cement floor. Between the outside walls of the house and the pantry are two thick inner walls." She had already moved a mattress and four gunnysacks of rice into the hallway by the pantry. Doyle also noticed that the living room windows were barricaded and piles of logs and a six-foot Union Jack was draped over a bookcase. "I know the Communists don't like a display of foreign flags," she told him, "but we just wanted to look at it."

Before Doyle left, she summoned her two servants, a smiling, white-jacketed No. 1 boy and a graying, gold-toothed *amah*. "Here," she explained, "are Lao Wu and Amah. Lao Wu has been in the family for forty-five years, Amah for thirty-four. What would they do if we ran away and left them?"

White Russians were the only people running away en masse. As part of our "Last Days of Shanghai" essay, we photographed some six thousand of them milling around the International Refugee Organization's headquarters seeking help. They had become an important part of the Shanghai community, building churches, schools, and clubs. Yet, they feared the Communists would send them back to Russia. At first, the IRO couldn't get any country to accept them. Finally, the Philippine government granted almost all who wanted to come temporary refuge on Samar Island.

The White Russians were first being vetted by Philippine Consul General Mariano Ezpeleta. Many, he told me, claimed they were aristocrats, listing their occupations as "Prince" or "Countess." He described how Countess Alexandra, who drove to the consulate in a chauffeured limousine and appeared before him festooned with jewels and wearing a mink coat despite the balmy spring weather, lived in a beautiful villa in Shanghai. But she couldn't abide the thought of staying on under the Communists. "Those awful people," she said. "I fled from them thirty years ago." The few Russians who were being denied sanctuary on Samar, Ezpeleta said, were desperados and gangsters wanted in several European capitals.

Birns and I spent several more days down on the docks interviewing and photographing the crowds of Russians as they camped there waiting for rusty old Chinese freighters to ferry them to safety.

Hardly anyone, especially the Russians, believed the Nationalists would really fight to keep Shanghai. All of their military preparations were considered part of a face-saving demonstration. Americans took comfort in the presence of a U.S. Navy armada, even though it had moved twenty miles north of Shanghai to an anchorage in Woosung, where the Huangpu flows into the Yangtze. The armada included the cruiser *St. Paul,* flagship of Vice Admiral Oscar Badger, commander of the U.S. Naval Forces in the Western Pacific; the destroyer *Duncan;* the troop transport *Chilton,* serving as a floating barracks for a U.S. Marine detachment; the auxiliary communications vessel *El Dorado;* and the hospital ship *Repose,* on which several *Amethyst* survivors were still recovering. An American President Line passenger ship was also due to stop in Shanghai. Clearly, there was plenty of room aboard these vessels to evacuate the entire American community—provided anyone wanted to leave.

Martial law was finally declared in Shanghai, providing more fodder for our photo essay. Sand-bagged sentry posts were erected at main intersections, armored cars rumbled through the streets, and Nationalist soldiers brandishing rifles poked their bayonets into the bundles of anyone entering the city, looking for hidden weapons. All exit roads from the city were choked with fleeing Chinese carrying what possessions they could on their backs. Censorship was enforced for the first time. When the censors killed a three-column story on the front page of the *Shanghai Evening Post and Mercury,* the editor, Gould, left the space blank, infuriating the censors and alarming his readers, who wondered what dire news had been deleted.

We foreign correspondents also began facing censorship problems. Associated Press bureau chief Fred Hampson succeeded in getting one unflattering story about the generalissimo past the censors by using General

Stilwell's description of him as the Peanut. Reynolds Packard, the colorful United Press Correspondent whose large Chinese lady-friend was known as the Manchu Monster, tried using the U.S. army nickname "Chancre Jack," for Chiang Kai-shek, but that didn't work. I was lucky, because many of my reports traveled to our editorial offices in New York in film packets, thus circumventing the censors.

Government officials were beginning to drift away, heading for Taiwan or Hong Kong. Mayor K. C. Wu, a Princeton graduate and always a highly quotable source, had turned over the municipal government reins to General Chen Liang—but not before he had entrusted parts of the mayor's archives, including selected intelligence files, to the Americans for safekeeping. Replacement Mayor Liang immediately proclaimed a citywide Health Week, and issued a decree ordering people to plant victory gardens to supply Shanghai with fresh vegetables. He, too, quickly departed. Again, Gould, never one to be cowed by the censors, wrote in his newspaper, "The mayor certainly was sincere. He found out what seemed best for his own health and promptly did it."

A few wealthy Chinese, I discovered, had been plotting for Shanghai to give up without a fight. Even gangster "Big Ears" Du Yuesheng, whose Green Gang had helped Chiang Kai-shek massacre thousands of Communists in 1927, contacted the Communist underground to say that he would do whatever possible to make it unnecessary for the People's Liberation Army to take Shanghai by force. Then he took off for Hong Kong. Du's plan, I learned, was to pay off the defending Nationalist generals in gold bars. The plot might have succeeded if Chiang Kai-shek hadn't unexpectedly appeared in Shanghai in late April and, in a nationwide radio address, announced, "There will be no surrender. Shanghai will fight to the end."

14

A CORRUPT REGIME'S CRUEL FINALE

In the absence of any detectable fighting, Birns and I continued looking for the "stark" and "gutsy" pictures our editors in New York were clamoring for. By early May, we didn't have to look very hard. As Shanghai went through its dying convulsions, residents were given a gruesome show every morning, and sometimes an even more gruesome matinee.

The show started with a mock trial in the courtyard of the central police station on Fuzhou Road. Three or four accused looters, gold smugglers, or suspected Communist agents were herded in to face the rump tribunal. Beneath a large Nationalist flag sewn to a somber black cloth, they stood and listened to a policeman recite their crimes, which were also spelled out in large Chinese characters painted on long-handled wooden paddles. Nobody, it appeared, was ever found innocent.

Quickly convicted, the doomed men (women were spared from this ordeal) were handed pen and paper to scratch out a will. Then, with their arms bound behind them and with the paddles wedged between their rope bindings so everybody could read what terrible crimes they had committed, the victims were loaded into an open truck for a slow ride around Shanghai. Thousands of silent onlookers lined every block to watch them pass. Of course, that was the purpose of this grisly parade, to make a spectacle of a few scapegoats, and keep the rest of the population in check. "The looting that wrecked Nanjing will not be tolerated here," announced the police chief.

After arriving at Zhabei Park, behind the railway station, the condemned men were shoved out of the truck, stood up against a bamboo fence, and shot point-blank through the back of the head. At least that's the way the executions had been described to me by the Chinese reporters taken along as witnesses, the foreign press having been barred from attending the actual executions.

After covering several mock trials, Birns and I felt obliged to ask for permission to complete the photographic sequence by following one group of victims to their death. Surprisingly, the police chief agreed to let us go along. I wish he hadn't.

On this particular afternoon, three purported Communist agents were loaded into the back of an old-style "black Mariah" instead of a truck. The cops told us to climb in with them. With the siren wailing and the doomed men screaming for mercy, we circled Shanghai. Peering out through the police van's wire grille at the huge gawking crowds, I felt like a caged animal going to my own slaughter.

At Zhabei Park, Jack handed me a Rolleiflex, "You shoot with this and I'll use the Contax," he said. Shoot was the wrong word. I was already verging on nausea. While working for UNRRA I had shot a number of picture stories on my own and was quite expert in handling a camera. Now, I was ready to plead my ineptness and let Jack photograph the whole bloody scene himself.

The cops wasted no time. They lined the men up a few feet apart. One cop held a revolver in his outstretched hand, leveling the barrel at the back of the first victim's head. As I peered down at the ground glass of the Rollei and adjusted the focusing knob, the executioner and his prey appeared as small images, even though they were standing only a few feet away. Better than seeing them through naked eyes, I thought.

Click! The victim froze at the sound of the trigger as the revolver failed to fire. So did I. It was a terrible moment for the cop, too, it suddenly occurred to me. At least with a whole firing squad doing the dirty work, nobody can tell if one gun misfires or who fired the fatal shot.

Another policeman jumped forward and let loose a quick burst with his Tommy gun. Blood spurted from the man's mouth as he crumpled onto the ground. The first cop then bent down and delivered the coup de grace. This time there was no chilling click. The revolver fired. But it didn't matter. The man was already dead.

For a second, while I cranked the handle of the camera to advance the film, I thought I'd forgotten to press the shutter button. So what if I missed the picture? *Life's* audience wouldn't be any poorer. And, as the reporter, I wouldn't have had to grope for words to describe this butchery.

By the time I'd refocused the Rollei, it was the second victim's turn. Another executioner stepped forward, pointing a carbine at the man's back. The macabre notion that the cops were using different weapons to give our pictures a little variety crossed my mind. I watched the executioner switch the gun onto automatic. Then the rapid-fire crack of his carbine rang in my ears.

Through the camera's ground glass, I saw the victim pitch forward and fall. No spurting blood this time. Studying the contact prints after they'd been air-expressed back to us from New York, I saw that the Rollei's fast shutter had caught the speeding bullet precisely as it was exiting from the victim's body. I could tell because the man's sweater was stretched to a sharp point out in front of his chest just before the bullet pierced the threads.

All this time, the third victim stood perfectly still, stoically waiting for the searing explosion that would be his last conscious moment. He was neatly dressed in black trousers and a white short-sleeve shirt. He never flinched. The tall wooden paddle proclaiming his crime stuck between his two bound hands never quivered. The man either had no nerves or he'd been drugged.

Another cop, much younger than his comrades, came forward like a rookie batter stepping up to the plate from the on-deck circle but brandishing a snub-nosed "grease gun" instead of a Louisville Slugger. He planted his feet in an open stance behind his target. Slowly, he raised the weapon and sighted down the short barrel, aiming between the shoulders of the white shirt.

I held my breath to steady the camera, expecting to hear the gun chatter. What's he waiting for? I wondered. Too scared to pull the trigger?

A shouted command came from behind me, and the chattering erupted—ten, twelve, fourteen shots before it finally stopped. The figure with the white shirt toppled backward, falling on the wooden paddle still wedged behind his hands. Slowly, the clean white shirt turned crimson. Would I ever be able to blot out the memory of this brutal scene? Would these killings be commemorated by the Communists sometime in the future, or have these three men died in vain? Is this the legacy Chiang Kai-shek wants to leave? Those questions were whirling through my brain as my stomach began to wretch.

On our way back to the bureau, Birns and I stopped in at the Palace Hotel for a couple of slugs of whisky. I felt both sick and angry that we had given those cops the satisfaction of photographing their savagery, even though I realized they were just carrying out orders. A little tipsy, I felt like sounding off to my bosses in New York when we finally reached the office. And I eagerly did.

"Bearing witness to these killings," I cabled *Life*'s managing editor, "is not the work of a reporter, but of a sacrificial priest."

Actually, I think I was mad at myself for having felt compelled to cover the executions. A secondhand report would have sufficed. And, feeling that way, I wanted to express that thought to the person who would soon be deciding whether or not to inflict those pictures on the eyes of the public.

"It took about one minute at today's executions to make me forget I'd ever had that breather with you folks back in New York," my cable continued. "The reason will be clear, I believe, after you've developed these rolls of film. The scenes of incomprehensible cruelty that you will see were committed by a regime that has already been stripped of its power. Even Harry Luce recognized that fact when we had lunch. In a few days Shanghai will be lost. Since the killings were pointless, doesn't that make publishing these pictures pointless, too?"

I ended the cable by saying, "I'll be curious to learn of your decision." The managing editor didn't reply. But he opted not to run the pictures.

I was still upset when I left the office, the executioners' shots and angry words of my cable still ringing in my ears. Fortunately, there was a wingding of a social event already planned for that evening to help calm me down. George Vine and his wife Ellen were throwing what I assumed was a "farewell to Shanghai" party on the roof garden of the Foreign Correspondents' Club. George and I had become good friends. Our Time–Life office occupied the third floor of the building belonging to the *North China Daily News,* of which George was editor, so we saw each other almost every day I was in town. A few weeks earlier, he and another British journalist had been arrested by the Nationalist secret police and threatened with execution for leaking a report on where the Communists planned to cross the Yangtze. The party was also to celebrate George's release.

While the festivities were going on inside, I remember standing out on the terrace atop Broadway Mansions and looking down at Suzhou Creek below. The sampans were still packed together so tightly you could barely see the filthy water keeping them afloat. The little boats looked just the same as they did when I first arrived in Shanghai three years before. Smoke curled from cook stoves in the stern. Babies tethered to the masts, crawled around the decks, appearing like small bugs from seventeen stories up. The next morning, the sampans were all gone, a sure sign that Shanghai, too, would soon be gone.

The Vines' party was the last to be held at the Foreign Correspondents' Club. We decided to close the club because the cooks and waiters were becoming sullen and aggressive. We didn't realize they had already been indoctrinated by Communist infiltrators and had formed a Broadway Mansions Collective. Also, all of the club's possessions, including its furniture, a Hammond organ, and two cars that were rented out with drivers to visiting correspondents, had been sold right after the party, the funds being used to relocate the club in Hong Kong.

By mid-May, anti-Communist propaganda had been turned up full blast. Paraders marched up and down the Bund waving Nationalist flags, while ogreish portraits of Mao blossomed on storefronts bearing the empty threat, "Shanghai will be his graveyard." At the same time, the foreign diplomats pleaded with garrison commander General Tang Enbo to declare Shanghai an open city. He refused to listen. "We will fight to our last drop of blood," he declared, a sure sign the situation was desperate. By then, Chiang had slipped away as unexpectedly as he had come. For a while, he had remained in the harbor aboard the cruiser *Taikang*. But without notice the ship hauled anchor and sailed leisurely down the South China coast before heading across the Taiwan Strait to the island fortress he had established.

Mao didn't want his troops to fight their way into the city. On the other hand, he was unwilling to allow the Nationalists a propaganda victory by letting them hold out too long against the overwhelming Communist force. Most Shanghai residents knew the Nationalist cause was hopeless as they watched the perimeter around the city rapidly shrink. They feared a prolonged defense would bring nothing but pillage and destruction. But a few optimists clung to the notion that, after a hundred years of foreign influence, the Western powers might finally intercede and prevent a Communist takeover. Some even argued that the Communists needed Shanghai to conduct their international business and, therefore, would maintain the great metropolis as a free-trade zone. "If the Communists are welcomed by conservative business interests, not to mention the general populace, it will not be surprising," declared Consul General Cabot in a dispatch to the State Department.

Not many of the correspondents, however, wanted to risk being trapped in Shanghai. Bob Doyle, my *Time* magazine counterpart, was one of the few who decided to stay on under the Communists, hoping to file exclusive eyewitness reports on the new regime. His decision proved to be a bad one. After being held virtually incommunicado for almost three months, he was finally expelled from Shanghai, only to be killed by bandits a short time later on an anthropological assignment in Indonesia.

Most of the correspondents had either left or were rapidly making plans to evacuate. Birns and I flew off to Taiwan on May 22, figuring the city was about to fall. Then, when it didn't, we flew back on a plane loaded to the ceiling with ammunition. We heard stories of many residents whose plans also kept shifting as the Communists failed to appear. Sue Crouch, a pretty Australian woman and former UNRRA colleague, had been counting on a June wedding. But with the Communists suddenly threatening Shanghai, she advanced the date to May 22. New invitations were mailed out, a wedding dress quickly stitched together, and a towering wedding cake baked. Then, on the eve of her wedding, she was warned that the Communists were expected to enter Shanghai the next day. The minister offered to marry her and her fiancé that night, but she insisted on taking a chance and waiting. Fortunately, the Communists didn't show up and the wedding proceeded as planned, attended by 150 friends.

On May 23, city officials were still holding victory parades and daily executions were still being carried out when apartment dwellers in the French Concession reported hearing the first sharp bursts of machine-gun fire coming from the southwest. Also, in Woosung to the north, at the juncture of the Huangpu and Yangtze rivers, where most of the foreign ships had found refuge, plumes of black smoke darkened the sky. Still, the local authorities claimed the situation was under control and that the city's inner defenses could not be breached. "Streets all bedecked by order to celebrate glorious Nationalist victory. Most shops open, police on job," Consul General Cabot cryptically noted in his diary.

Actually, the Communist attack was being launched on the grounds of The Limit, where Billy and Gladys Hawkings were still holding out in their home. They heard a loud banging on the door and sent their old servant, Lau Wu, to see who was there. A Communist messenger handed him a note ordering the Hawkings to move out. But they stayed, trapped in their dwelling while shells whistled overhead. When the firing stopped, Gladys opened the door and called out in Chinese to three People's Liberation Army soldiers. They looked startled at this *gweilo* ("a person with round eyes," the slang term for occidentals) addressing them in impeccable Chinese. "No," the soldiers said politely. "We don't want to billet our men in your house." Then he smiled and insisted on shaking Gladys' hand.

The next day, every road into Shanghai was clogged with retreating Nationalist soldiers. Some marched in parade formation. Others, caked with mud from the battlefield, streaked through the city in terror and confusion. A few stragglers yanked civilians from their bicycles and pedicabs, or grabbed anything they could carry from the arms of the petrified owners.

At midnight on May 24, Communist infantrymen commanded by General Chen Yi began filtering into the city through the French Concession. They moved as quietly as they could. In small groups they advanced slowly down the sidewalks of Avenue Joffre, tying their mules and horses to storefronts and sidling close to the buildings for protection against fire from any Nationalist snipers in the surrounding apartment buildings.

The Communists' mustard-colored uniforms were clean and the men well armed with Bren guns and Tommy guns. Hand grenades hung from their belts, bandoleers of cartridges from their shoulders. At every halt, they slumped on the sidewalk to rest.

Along Nanjing Road, Shanghai's main business street, the Communists herded captured Nationalists into gas stations and stores. When an angry crowd of civilians turned on a frightened Nationalist soldier, Red troops dispersed them. At one busy corner, a Communist noncom stood guard over a lone Nationalist soldier squatting in a doorway. "What about him?" asked a passerby. "He's very happy now," replied the noncom. The soldier, puffing a cigarette given to him by his captor, grinned sheepishly.

Most of the Communists were peasant boys, clearly more amazed at Shanghai than Shanghai was at them. They gawked at the fancy hotels and movie palaces. "What day is it?" asked one. "We've been walking and fighting for a week."

Finally, by 9:00 A.M. on May 25, the conquering troops reached the main business district. They took over the central police station and city hall and raided what was left of the archives. "Have the Communists really come?" asked a civilian onlooker. *"Balu laile"* ("the Communists have come"), replied an officer.

Within an hour, Shanghai turned out to celebrate. A hastily thrown-up banner near the American Club proclaimed: WELCOME TO THE PEOPLE'S LIBERATION ARMY. Red flags were draped over doorways, and truckloads of students careened through the streets, jubilantly waving pennants.

From loudspeakers all over town, Communist songs blared above the distant rattle of machine guns. One popular song went:

Reactionaries who exploit the people deserve to be cut into a thousand
pieces.
Big landlords, big warlords, big compradors, big families, all conspire
together.
Therefore, we poor people suffer.

Although Garrison Commander Tang Enbo had flown the coop, some of his troops were still putting up rear-guard resistance, firing from sandbagged emplacements along the Suzhou Creek in front of the Broadway Mansions. Almost all of the correspondents had vacated the building. But Margaret Hampson was still there, telephoning minute-by-minute eyewitness reports to her husband, Fred, at the Associated Press headquarters in Frenchtown.

Nationalist snipers atop Broadway Mansions were also shooting indiscriminately down at the street below even though many of the nearby shops had already reopened, as had the Central Post Office two blocks away. Letter carriers could be seen exiting from the massive old structure, starting on their regular morning rounds.

The few foreigners trapped in the Broadway Mansions were terrified that the Communists would start shelling the building. But after holding out for two days, the defending Nationalist soldiers realized that the Communists had crossed to the north bank farther up the Suzhou Creek and outflanked them. Only then were they persuaded to hoist a white flag. Their officers issued them red armbands to wear as they finally left the building. The price of surrender, it turned out, was a sumptuous farewell lunch prepared by the Foreign Correspondents' Club chef.

The tawdry Red Light District in Hongkew, behind Broadway Mansions, was packed with fleeing Nationalist deserters. Most of them had already tossed their weapons into the Huangpu River and were desperately hunting down shops selling used clothing they could change into. Soon, the streets were strewn with discarded uniforms, a bonanza for the army of ill-clad beggars who knew they would never be mistaken for Nationalist soldiers.

Later, it occurred to me that most of that used clothing probably came from the U.S. courtesy of my former employer, UNRRA, just as many of the American weapons thrown away by the fleeing soldiers had come from our war surplus arsenals in the Philippines, where I had served in the army. The guns had proven useless. But the used clothing, even in the final hours of the civil war, was still serving a good purpose.

Had I supervised the unloading of any of that clothing when it arrived in Shanghai? I wondered. Could one of those discarded rifles have been the one I toted in Manila? From the day I landed in Shanghai in1946, I had felt closely connected to China's civil war. And the connection was still strong as I reported on the last-minute acts of desperation by the defeated Nationalist soldiers. The civil war sputtered on for several months while the Communists mopped up in the south. But, essentially, it was over with the fall of Shanghai. Yet, I knew my own involvement would never end.

As the remnants of Chiang's armies headed for the scores of Nationalist ships waiting off the coast at Woosung, pitched battles continued to erupt here and there. In Pudong, across the river from Shanghai, what was left of one Nationalist infantry division confiscated thousands of sacks of sugar awaiting shipment on a wharf to use in place of sandbags for protecting their gun emplacements. That enterprising last-ditch defense effort proved to be futile, just as almost every defensive move made by Chiang Kai-shek's armies had since the start of the war. Another Nationalist division farther down the river had already defected, leaving those troops in Pudong stranded behind their wall of sugar.

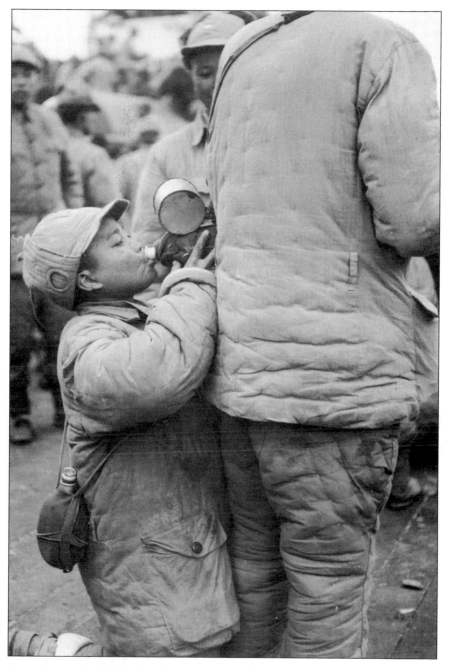

Young boys, called "little devils," ran messages and performed odd chores around infantry campsites. Occasionally the army issued them rifles and pressed them into action as combatants. JACK BIRNS, COURTESY OF LIFE.

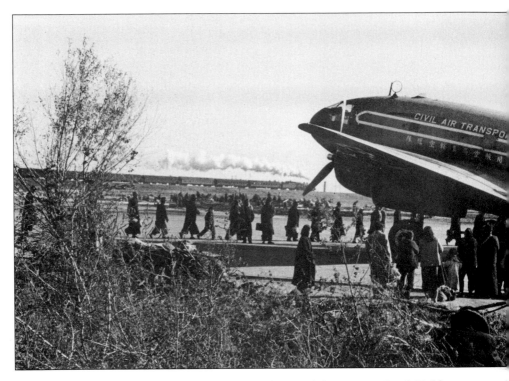

Civilians fleeing Mukden in October 1948 patiently waited their turn at South Field to board one of the hundred evacuation flights a day to Tianjin, Qingdao, and Beijing. The pilots of the three civilian airlines, CAT, CNAC, and CATC, logged sixty hours a week during this emergency operation. JACK BIRNS, COURTESY OF LIFE.

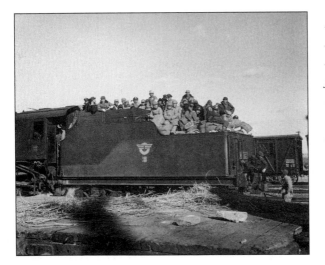

Nationalist soldiers fleeing Mukden who couldn't squeeze into or atop the freight cars took their place in the coal pile of a steam locomotive's tender. From a distance, the author noted, their yellow-padded uniforms made the engine and long string of boxcars look like sausage links covered with mustard. JACK BIRNS, COURTESY OF LIFE.

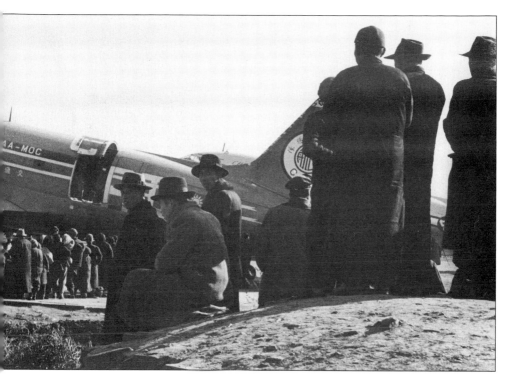

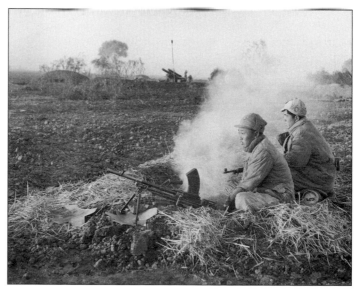

Two machine-gunners of the highly touted Nationalist 207th infantry division burned a fire to cut Mukden's early morning chill. Practically all of the members of this division were either killed or captured the following day.
JACK BIRNS,
COURTESY OF LIFE.

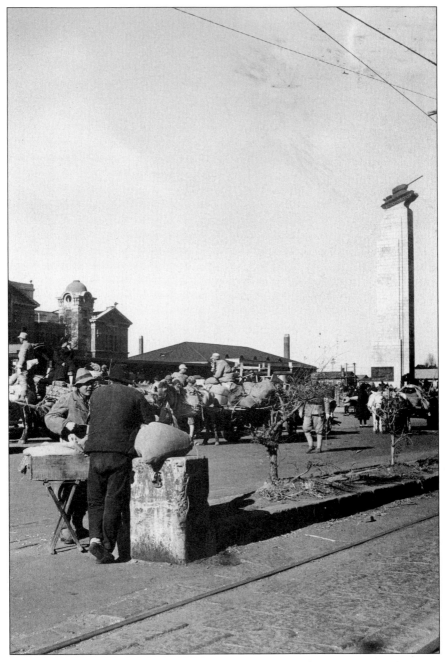

*Although all of the passenger trains departing Mukden's railyard were already filled
with escaping soldiers, a crowd of would-be ticket buyers wedged themselves between
the depot and the 100-foot-high Russian World War II victory obelisk topped with a
Soviet tank.* JACK BIRNS, COURTESY OF LIFE.

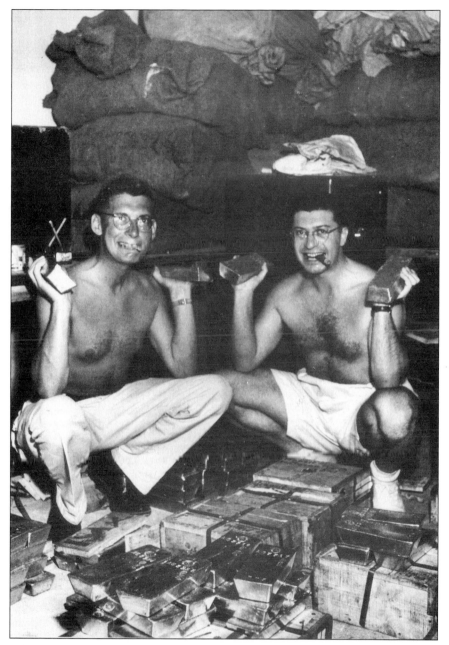

The author (left) and photographer Jack Birns with a pile of 400-Troy-ounce gold bricks in a Macao smuggling sydicate's basement foundry. Operators smelted the gold into ten-ounce bars, then hid them aboard junks destined for the black market in Shanghai and other China ports where the Nationalist currency had become virtually worthless. JACK BIRNS, COURTESY OF LIFE.

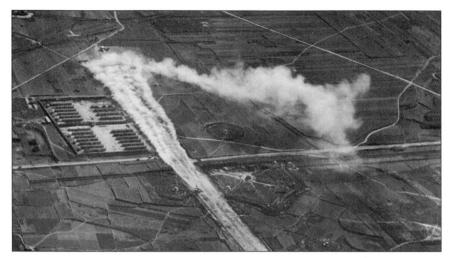

Plumes of dust followed a CAT plane after making a quick landing and takeoff on an improvised dirt airstrip in besieged Taiyuan. Communist mortars honeycombed the surrounding hills around the strip, and most of the planes participating in the $300,000-a-day airlift had to parachute rice and ammo in order to keep Marshal Yan Xishan's capital city alive. JACK BIRNS, COURTESY OF LIFE.

This lone Nationalist soldier was shouting to the men occupying a pillbox in the no-man's-land outside Taiyuan. Yan's 90,000 defenders included Nationalist troops, mercenary Japanese soldiers left over from World War II, and his own private army. JACK BIRNS, COURTESY OF LIFE.

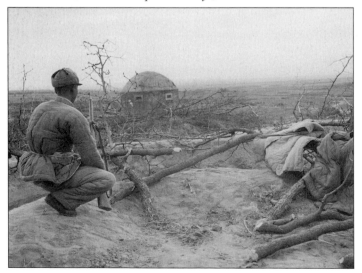

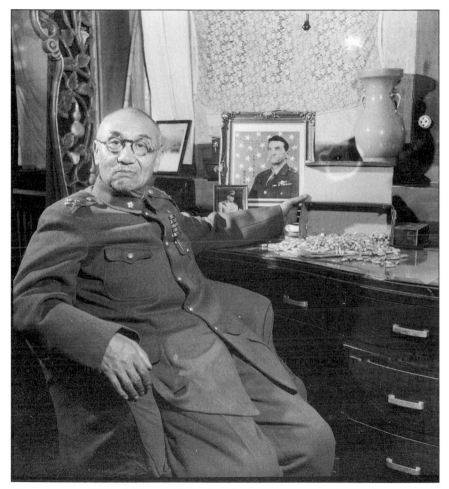

Sixty-six-year-old Yan Xishan with five hundred potassium cyanide capsules spread across his desk. He and his five hundred commanders vowed to commit suicide if the Communists captured Taiyuan. Yan also promised to spread gasoline around his office and set it afire before swallowing the poison so the Communists wouldn't find his body. The old marshal did neither, but followed Chiang Kai-shek to Taiwan where he died of a heart attack in 1960. Adorning his desk is a picture of his hero, General Claire Chennault, the former Flying Tiger commander who later founded CAT.
JACK BIRNS, COURTESY OF LIFE.

*A soldier in the Nationalists'
13th Army Group as he
catnapped beside his tank in
the heavily-fortified village of
Zhouzhuang during the
million-man Battle of the
Huai-Hai in November 1948.
His tank corps swung into action
the next morning in a failed
attempt to wrest a nearby
village from the Communists.*
JACK BIRNS, COURTESY OF LIFE.

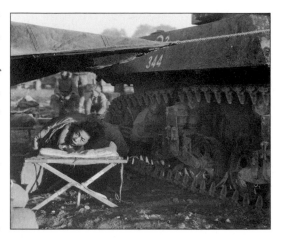

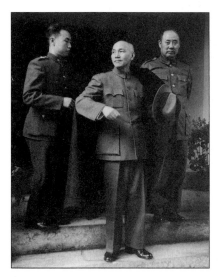

*Chiang Kai-shek (center)
donned a cape and left
hurriedly after our interview.
General Fu Zuoyi (right)
would later surrender Beijing
and defect to the Communists.*
JACK BIRNS, COURTESY OF LIFE.

*General Li Mi, commander of the 13th Army
Group and one of Chiang Kai-shek's most capable
generals, served under U.S. General Joseph
Stilwell, during World War II. In this photo he
was wearing a private's uniform to make it
difficult for the Communists to identify him in
the event of his capture. After the Communists
won the Battle of the Huai-Hai, Li escaped to
Burma with some of his troops. From there they
continued to make armed forays into China.*
JACK BIRNS, COURTESY OF LIFE.

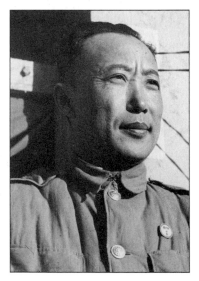

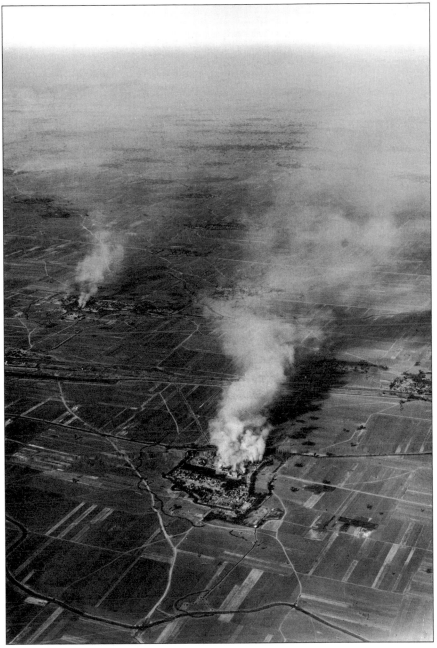

The Nationalists' 13th Army Group shelled many Communist-held villages during the height of the Battle of the Huai Hai. The surviving remnants of the Nationalist armies finally surrendered on January 10, 1949, opening the way for the Communists to attack Nanjing and Shanghai. JACK BIRNS, *COURTESY OF* LIFE.

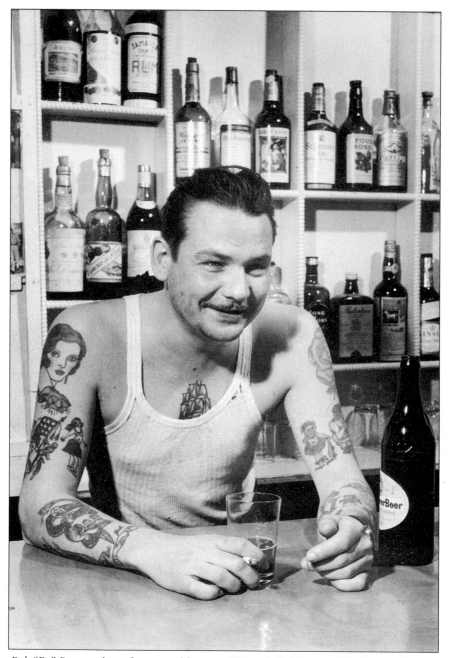

Bob "Bo" Brown, thirty-four-year-old owner of Shanghai's Diamond Bar, became his own best customer as business faded away with the approach of the Communists in early May 1949. A merchant sailor from Chicago, Brown jumped ship in 1946 to buy the waterfront dive. One of his American competitors claimed a year earlier he'd been offered $40,000 for his bar. "Now," he said, "I couldn't give it away." JACK BIRNS, COURTESY OF LIFE.

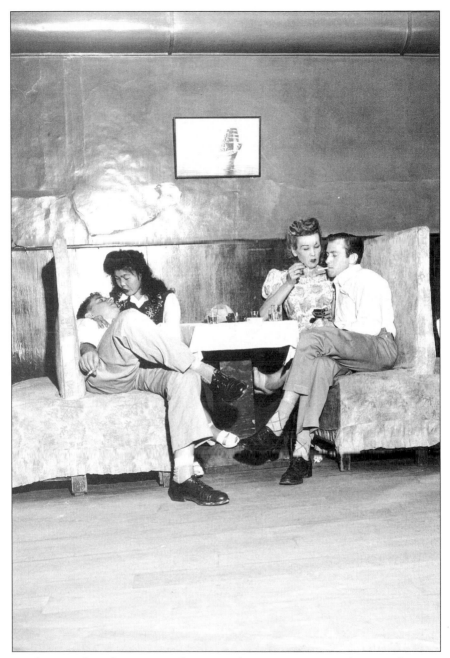

A Chinese and a White Russian "hostess" in the American Bar, another waterfront dive, as they tried to persuade two U.S. merchant sailors to forget Shanghai's 10 P.M. curfew and stay ashore with them for the night. The curfew was finally imposed after the Communists attacked two British warships on the Yangtze River, 140 miles from Shanghai. JACK BIRNS, COURTESY OF LIFE.

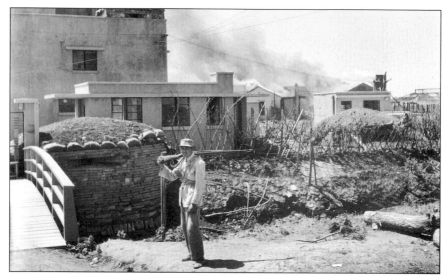

The Nationalist Army cut down trees and burned down buildings to clear a field of fire for their heavy artillery as the Communists approached Shanghai in mid-May 1949. But when the Red Army units finally arrived at this spot a week later, the defending troops fled. JACK BIRNS, COURTESY OF LIFE.

Even though the Communists had already reached the outskirts of Shanghai, Nationalist units continued to hold close-order drill atop the garage next to the Broadway Mansions, where all of the foreign correspondents were billeted. This photo was taken from the author" bedroom window. JACK BIRNS, COURTESY OF LIFE.

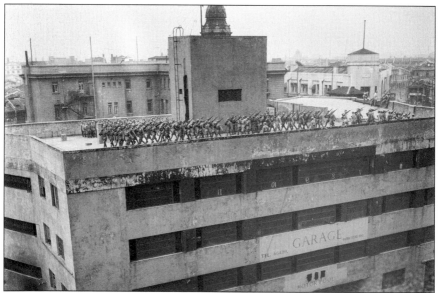

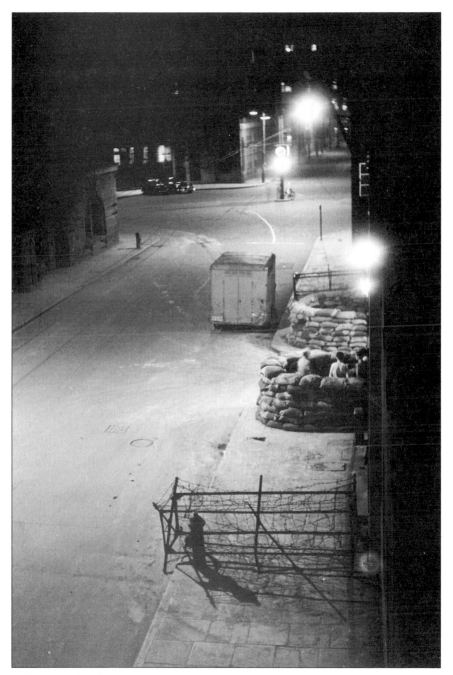

Officials declared martial law and set up barricades in Shanghai's main thoroughfares to guard the deserted streets during curfew hours. But nobody believed the Nationalists would stand and fight, even though General Tang Enbo, entrusted with the city's defense, declared: that "Shanghai will be China's Stalingrad." JACK BIRNS, COURTESY OF LIFE.

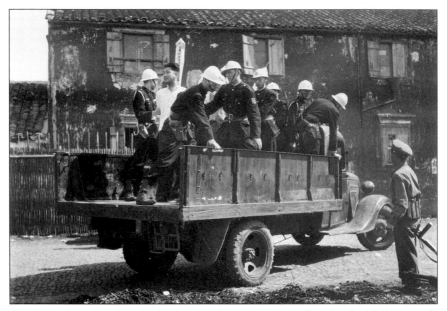

Hoping to keep discipline in the threatened city, police gave drumhead trials to accused black marketers and suspected Communist agents. Then they trucked the accused through the streets on the way to their execution. The doomed man in the white shirt has a signboard sticking up proclaiming his crime. JACK BIRNS, COURTESY OF LIFE.

Police lined up the victims in Zhabei Park behind the railroad station and shot them one by one. The white-shirted man lying on the ground endured a horrible moment when the executioner's revolver failed to fire. Another policeman let loose a quick burst with his Tommy Gun, although the cop with the revolver continued to pump bullets into the dead man. JACK BIRNS, COURTESY OF LIFE.

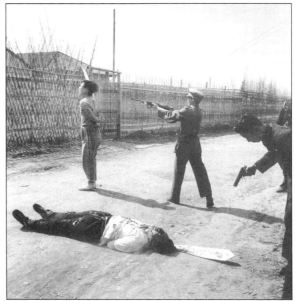

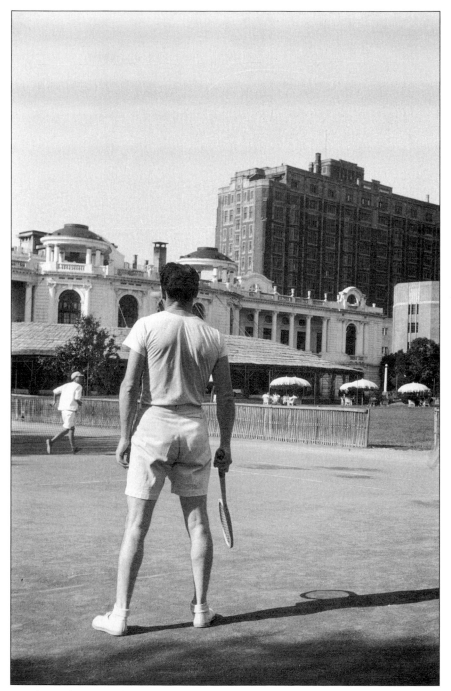

Residents of the French concession, like those seen here still playing tennis at Le Cercle Sportif, seemed unperturbed as Shanghai was about to fall. JACK BIRNS, COURTESY OF LIFE.

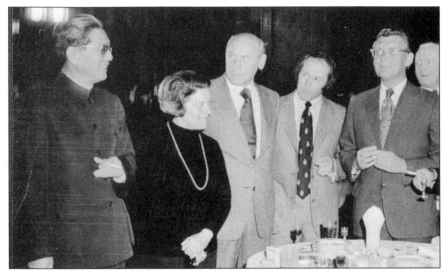

During the 1973 reception for Princess Ida of Ethiopia at the Great Hall of the People in Beijing, China's Deputy Foreign Minister Qiao Guanhua (left) bawls out the dismayed-looking author for his breach of protocol in presenting Premier Zhou Enlai with an album of old war pictures that Rowan had shot while working for CNRRA. Rowan hoped the album would encourage Zhou to invite him back to Henan Province where they had met briefly in 1947. AUTHOR PHOTO.

The author's wife, Helen, proved to be a western curiosity when the Rowans visited Kaifeng in 1981. After being rebuffed for giving Zhou the picture album, Rowan tried for eight years before being granted permission by China's Foreign Office to go back and write an article for Fortune *on the changes that had occurred in Henan since the war. On this return trip he visited and photographed all the villages that his trucks had delivered relief supplies to thirty-four years earlier. The sandy rutted roads had all been paved over, and the old city walls torn down. AUTHOR PHOTO.*

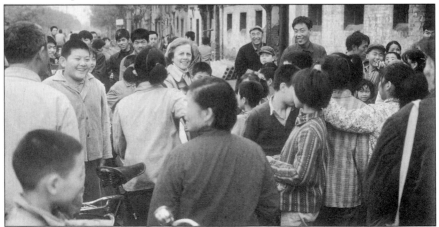

In the end, Mao allowed all Nationalist remnants in Shanghai to escape to their ships. Capturing them, he decided, was not worth causing further destruction to a city he already controlled. After all, the ultimate victory prize in his long, hard fight was not more Nationalist prisoners of war, but the country's throbbing commercial center, Shanghai—in the eyes of the world, the symbol of China.

Mao Zedong did not appear there to personally accept that victory prize until November. A month earlier, on a blustery October 1, riding through Beijing's Tiananmen Square in a captured American jeep, he had already proclaimed the founding of the People's Republic. "China has stood up," he proudly announced. "Never again will the Chinese be an enslaved people."

But Mao's belated arrival in Shanghai marked for most people there the true beginning of the new order. Although still apprehensive about what to expect, they nevertheless sang of his glory:

> *Chairman Mao can be compared to the sun in the east,*
> *Which shines over the world so brightly, so brightly,*
> *Heigh-ai-yo, heigh-heigh-heigh-yo,*
> *Without Chairman Mao how can there be peace?*
> *Heigh-ai-yo.*

This home-grown poet-philosopher from China's heartland had brought with him the myth of an unending class struggle. But he was also a practical man, and as tough as any warlord who preceded him. But, unlike them, he saw early on that the old order was crumbling under the weight of Western civilization. Chiang Kai-shek, he realized, had failed to build a solid base for Nationalist China. Chiang saw to it that it that his country had bombers before it had a good rail system, cars before bicycles, radios before decent telephone service. As Mao vowed to change those things, his speeches quoted everyone, from Thomas Jefferson to Friedrich Engels and Sun Yat-sen.

But Mao knew that changing China would cost many lives. "A revolution is no invitation to a banquet," he once declared. And his men followed loyally, fought fiercely, even died when asked to for what they hoped would be the end of tyranny. Yet, despite his strong ideology, Mao remained a genuine romantic, with the ability to arouse fervent popular devotion. That was his strength.

Chiang Kai-shek was perhaps just as strong a leader. But with a different vision for modernizing China, he never succeeded in arousing popular devotion. That was his failure. Without it, despite superior weapons, vast quantities of humanitarian aid, and billions of dollars from the United States, he lost China's civil war. And that loss would enable the "Great Helmsman," as Mao's followers called him, to change the world more than any man of his century.

When I flew out of Shanghai in May 1949, I assumed it was for the last time, that I would never see China again. Peering down at the city's vanishing skyline with the Huangpu River snaking through it, I was gripped by sadness, as if bidding a final farewell to a rollicking old friend.

Goodbye, amazing city, I thought. It wasn't just your clash between East and West and rich and poor that set you apart. Nor was it your sex and other vices, your casual everything-for-sale attitude, or your rampant violence and inbred corruption. It was your day-to-day excitement that will never be duplicated.

Flashing through my mind were the words of that misplaced missionary who cried out, "God owes an apology to Sodom and Gomorra if He lets Shanghai endure."

Silly preacher, they sent you to the wrong town. Shanghai, you were wonderful. No apologies needed. But you'll never be the same again—and neither will I.

I was right about that, but wrong about never going back, though it would be almost a quarter of a century before China opened up again to American reporters. Mao immediately slammed down the Bamboo Curtain, closing off the vast land to all Americans but a few Communist sympathizers, just as his mentors in the Kremlin had done with the Iron Curtain. So it was impossible back then to guess how drastically things might change. We Old China-hands (as we called ourselves despite our youth) could only assume that the changes wrought by Mao would be brutal. And, indeed, they were.

Once, while flying over the battlefields during the war, he had composed a poem describing how Genghis Khan and China's early rulers were uncultured. "These men belong to the past," he wrote. "Only today there are men of feeling." The Great Helmsman may have been a man of feeling, but he soon proved to be just as tyrannical as any emperor.

First, he consolidated his power by killing or destroying millions of class enemies. Even General Lin Biao, considered his most likely successor, died in a suspicious plane crash. Next came the Great Leap Forward of the late 1950s, during which tens of millions more people starved; then the Hundred Flowers Campaign, which decimated intellectual life; and finally the decade-long Cultural Revolution led by Mao's third wife, Jiang Qing. (His first wife, Yang Kaihui, the daughter of his revered school teacher, was executed by the Nationalists. His second wife, He Zizhen, fell mentally ill and was sent to the Soviet Union for treatment.) A former stage and screen star turned violent revolutionary, Jiang Qing and her "Gang of Four" radical cohorts began undermining the aging Mao, bringing China to the edge of chaos. Thousands of intellectuals were beaten to death or died from their injuries. Tried by a People's Court and condemned to death in 1976, her sentence was commuted to life under house arrest. She died in 1991.

We reporters, shut out of the mainland during most of this turmoil, were forced to cover what transpired there from Hong Kong or Taiwan as so-called "China-watchers." To do that, I moved the Time–Life bureau into the bridal suite of the posh Peninsula Hotel in Kowloon. For a mere $300 per month (today, that same suite costs $800 per day), it met our temporary needs perfectly. The living room became the office, the bedroom my home. There were plenty of spry young bellhops to whisk messages back and forth to the Cable and Wireless office, located in the ornate hangar-size lobby, where gold smugglers, arms traders, and other wheeler-dealers of the East conducted their nefarious business over afternoon tea.

Trying to peek through the Bamboo Curtain was frustrating, to say the least. We interviewed defectors and foreign travelers, relied on translators to monitor Communist broadcasts and newspapers, leaned heavily on the political officers at the Consulate General, and, above all, kept meticulous files. We even noted where party leaders stood in relation to Mao during their appearances atop the great gate of the Forbidden City. Still, it was almost impossible to keep track of the rise and fall and rise again of mercurial leaders like Deng Xiaoping, who was vilified one day and praised the next. So, at best, most of our reports filed from Hong Kong were highly speculative.

For a while, the chances appeared bleak that Mao's strict socialist state would ever relax its stranglehold on the people. Meanwhile, ultra-conservatives in the U.S., goaded by Senator Joseph McCarthy, went on a witch-hunt, pillorying the State Department's two most knowledgeable China experts, John Service and John Paton Davies, Jr. for the "loss of China," as if China was theirs to lose. How stunned those Red-baiting McCarthyites would be to learn that Mao's successors have come to embrace most of the concepts of capitalism—not only welcoming American investors with open arms, but with open wallets as well, for joint ventures. Or that Chinese cities once under attack by Mao's troops would become tourist meccas: containing luxury hotels, including Hyatts and Holiday Inns; haute couture boutiques owned by Ralph Lauren and Gucci; noisy karaoke bars; Kentucky Fried Chicken franchises; and the Communists' own so-called Friendship Stores, catering to the invading armies of foreign arts and crafts hunters. No, not in our wildest imaginings could even we, as experienced China-watchers, have envisioned such stunning changes.

Life's editors relieved me of that frustrating China-watching post in 1950 and sent me off to cover the Cold War in Europe, the Korean War, and finally the Vietnam War, interspersed with several reporting and editing assignments in the U.S. I also married Helen Rounds, a charming young *Life* picture researcher, and we started a family, that quickly grew to include four sons. Then, interrupting my Time Inc. career, I spent two entrepreneurial years launching a pair of magazines for seafront dwellers on the East Coast, *On the Sound* and *On the Shore*.

Rejoining the Luce empire as *Time*'s Hong Kong bureau chief in 1972, my first priority was to go back to China. By then, the Bamboo Curtain had opened a crack. American reporters still weren't welcome despite President Nixon's much-heralded meeting with Mao earlier that year supposedly paving the way for journalistic exchanges. But it took some fancy finagling and marathon flying to finally get to the mainland, only a subway ride away.

I started by badgering the Communist travel agency in Hong Kong, which kept losing my visa applications. Then one day, they informed me that Emperor Haile Selassie of Ethiopia was about to establish a commercial air link between Addis Ababa and Shanghai and Beijing. "You're a reporter. Why don't you request a seat on the inaugural flight," the head of the agency suggested.

It so happened that I had once interviewed the "King of Kings, Conquering Lion of Judah," as the wily old five-foot-four-inch Ethiopian emperor was known. He had invited me to lunch at his palace. At first, it appeared that it was I who was going to be lunch for a pair of hungry-looking lions flanking the palace gate. But, escorted safely inside past those two live, unchained beasts, the interview couldn't have gone more smoothly, especially since it was known that His Imperial Highness harbored deep suspicions of the foreign press. So I wired him for permission to join the official entourage on the inaugural flight that was being led by his granddaughter, Princess Ida. "Please be advised that a seat on our plane has been reserved for your magazine," the emperor's secretary wired back.

The logistics, nevertheless, proved incredibly complicated. It meant flying first to Bombay via Bangkok and picking up a loosely connecting flight to Addis, where a special Chinese visa was issued, then backtracking to Bombay on the new Ethiopian Airlines jet, which finally flew nonstop to Shanghai—or would have if weather hadn't diverted the plane to Guangzhou. So, after sixty-three hours and 11,565 miles of flying, I landed in China, exactly 111 miles from my starting point in Hong Kong. A few hours later, the weather cleared and we took off again for an overnight rest stop in Shanghai.

Arriving in Shanghai in February 1973 after a twenty-four-year absence, I was surprised to be there all right. But not surprised by the dullness of that once-vibrant metropolis. It was like encountering a roaring old reprobate who had survived a stroke. The physiognomy of the place was the same. But, drained of its color and slaked of its ardor, the once-wildest city in the world was barely staggering along under Communism.

The evening ride in from the airport was dismal. The city was dark, all of the flashy neon replaced by sickly, flickering yellow bulbs. The spell binding cacophony of the streets that kept me awake during my first nights in 1946 had evaporated, giving way to the muffled whirr of thousands of bicycle wheels. More telling now were the sparsely stocked store shelves, which spoke of the disastrous Cultural Revolution still in progress.

The center of Shanghai hadn't added one new building to its skyline, and many of the old ones appeared unoccupied. All the foreign banks and businesses, along with the *taipans* who ran them, had transferred their headquarters to Hong Kong. So had the wealthy Chinese. Even the once-teeming Huangpu River that I had patrolled up and down aboard a tug, keeping an eye on UNRRA's cargoes, appeared devoid of foreign ships.

I checked into the old Cathay Hotel, a block up the Bund from where the Time–Life office had been. Sadly, the plush establishment formerly owned by Sir Victor Sassoon had metamorphosed into the run-down, government-owned Peace Hotel. The two cheery doormen who used to hustle the suitcases of arriving guests into the art deco marble lobby had been replaced by a pair of stone-faced sentries armed with automatic rifles. And the reception desk, which used to be staffed with British-accented Chinese concierges in cutaways and striped pants, was now manned by men and women of the Hotel Revolutionary Committee, all dressed in black padded jackets and baggy pants.

When the Big Ben clock atop the old Customs House a few blocks away sounded the hour, I thought, At last something familiar. But no, Red Guards had changed the chimes to play "The East is Red," Communist China's national anthem. I could hardly wait to get out of the half-dead commercial capital. Mercifully, Princess Ida's entourage took off for Beijing the following morning, before all my well-preserved memories of Shanghai had been erased.

Flying north in her Boeing 707, there again was the vast beauty of old China—misty purple peaks marching off to meet the snowy Himalayas, the mighty Yellow and Yangtze rivers slithering like two dusty snakes across the dun-colored Central Plain, where my truck convoys had run, and finally, the ground turning a pale green as we swooped low over fields of winter cabbage growing right up to the edge of the runway of Beijing's airport.

Inside the terminal, a larger-than-life portrait of Mao beamed benevolently from the wall, accompanied by a few of his favorite quotations: PRACTICE MARXISM, NOT REVISIONISM, BE OPEN AND ABOVEBOARD, DO NOT INTRIGUE OR CONSPIRE. Did the Chairman really fear that newly arrived visitors might not be aboveboard and conspire and intrigue during their visit to his capital?

In any case, Mao was too old and ailing to play host to his newfound friends from Ethiopia. The official reception for Princess Ida was left to Zhou Enlai, the shrewd Communist negotiator who had dropped in unexpectedly at our UNRRA headquarters in Kaifeng. Now, almost singlehandedly, he was attempting to reestablish diplomatic and trade relations with the rest of the world, while anti-Western outbursts, led by bands of Red Guards continued at home.

We China-watchers in Hong Kong had been following Zhou's behind-the-scenes maneuverings with considerable awe. When extremists burned down the British Embassy, it was he who delivered the official apology. But then it was said that the suave premier, unlike his boss, Mao, "could put a cosmopolitan face on Chinese Communism," which he was now doing for Princess Ida and her Ethiopian delegation.

The main social event during our visit was a cocktail reception given by Zhou in the Great Hall of the People. The building's exterior appeared as a giant, gray concrete block anchored on the edge of Tiananmen Square. But the interior was breathtaking. A massive interior stairway swept upward from the entrance—"a marble glacier with a river of red carpeting cascading down its middle," I noted, and then added, "as cumulous clouds of crystal glittered in the chandeliers overhead." Waiting to greet his royal guests at the top of what seemed like a flight of neverending steps stood the premier, brisk and businesslike, and very trim in a plain gray tunic with matching gray trousers. A miniature red Chairman Mao button pinned to his tunic gave the only dash of color to his outfit. Could this be the scraggly bearded brigadier general who had sat across the dinner table from me in Kaifeng? Except for the dark piercing eyes peering out from beneath his bushy eyebrows, I would never have recognized him.

For the next two hours, Zhou moved systematically through the assembled throng, toasting and shaking hands with each visiting dignitary. His winsome, steely smile reminded me of *Taking Tiger Mountain by Strategy*, a Communist opera we had suffered through the night before, as guests of Madame Mao. The social strategy of the premier was obviously aimed at winning the hearts of the Ethiopians, and everyone else at the huge reception.

After each round of handshakes, a waiter gave the premier a moist washrag to wipe his hands. His right hand, I remembered him telling us in Kaifeng, had been injured during the Long March and was still sensitive. However, the washrag routine didn't slow down the good-natured give and take with his guests as he fielded their questions and answered them with a quip that evoked ripples of laughter.

"Are you coming to Ethiopia?" one guest asked the premier through his attractive female interpreter.

"I don't know which airline to take," replied Zhou.

"Sir, are you planning any trips abroad?"

"I have too many debts," he answered. "I'm going to let the foreign minister do the traveling." But when he tossed back his head and laughed, I noticed his eyes didn't give off the same gaiety they had years before.

Suddenly, there he was, the double-barreled boss of China's domestic and foreign policy, extending his hand to me.

"Your Excellency, I have something for your archives." Then I handed Zhou the gift-wrapped album I had brought with me from Hong Kong. It contained some fifty enlargements of photographs I had taken in 1947, while convoying UNRRA supplies to the Communist villages south of the Yellow River.

Zhou looked perplexed, reluctant to take my gift. The Communists, I knew, had reservations about accepting anything that smacked of cumshaw. That became apparent while checking out of the Peace Hotel in Shanghai when the room boy chased me all the way down to the lobby with a worn-out razor blade that I had discarded in the bathroom. He mistook it for a gift.

Finally, Zhou's interpreter took the package for him. I explained what was in it and added that the premier's and my paths had crossed briefly in Henan Province.

"That was years ago during the War of Liberation," I said, using the Communists' term for China's civil war.

Zhou nodded. He seemed to understand what was being said even before it was translated. Then he raised his glass of *Mao Tai* and touched it to mine. *"Gambei,"* he said before drifting away to the next group of guests.

Evidently, my gift to the premier was a faux pas of the first order. A few minutes later, Qiao Guanhua, the deputy foreign minister, rushed over and asked for an explanation of my bad behavior. No breach of protocol was intended, I assured him. My only purpose in presenting the album was the hope that the old pictures might elicit an invitation from the premier for me to revisit Henan.

"That's not possible," said the deputy foreign minister. "Perhaps some other time," he added, his scowl changing into a smile. As things turned out, an invitation to go back and report on the changes in the province was finally extended to me eight years later. By then, I had already made a second trip back to China. But it was never clear if it was the old photos that had done the trick.

My second trip took place in 1975, accompanying President Jerry Ford to Beijing for his meeting with Mao. When Ford was vice president, my wife and I had been invited to dinner with him and Betty. Then, after he became president, I had interviewed him in the White House for a book about the rescue of the American container ship *Mayaguez,* captured by the Cambodians. So *Time* sent me along hoping that my personal access as a friend might produce some interesting insights about what surely would be the last meeting between Chairman Mao and an American president. In fact, Mao had become so feeble that the Chinese government had only reluctantly given in to Secretary of State Henry Kissinger's prodding for the meeting, considered of vital importance to Ford, with the U.S. election just a year away.

Right from the start of the state banquet at the Great Hall of the People, I could feel the cool reception being given the president. This time, substituting as host for the ailing Mao and for Zhou who was also ill, was First Vice Premier Deng Xiaoping, well known to us China-watchers for his lack of charm and manners. Even Kissinger referred to him as that "nasty little man." Aside from his blunt talk, Deng had a habit at affairs like this of spitting noisily into a spittoon placed by his side. "You must forgive me," he'd say. "I'm just a country boy."

Today, Deng is widely acclaimed for his leadership in modernizing China and for bringing it into the twenty-first century. But at the time of Ford's visit his reputation was still shaky. The following year, as the Cultural Revolution came to a climax, he was publicly excoriated for being "a high-living potentate who used his office to indulge his gluttonous tastes" and for his "bourgeois devotion to Mah-Jongg and bridge." For those sins, Red Guards labeled him a "capitalist roader" and paraded him through the streets of Beijing with a dunce cap pulled down over his ears. But Deng was a tough political cat with many lives. One of his favorite sayings was, "It doesn't matter if a cat is white or black as long as it catches mice."

From off in the distance, where the press corps was seated, we could barely see the diminutive five-foot-four-inch-tall vice premier. Even when he stood up to give the ceremonial toasts, we could only see his upraised glass. But the edge in his voice was clearly discernible as he criticized Ford's and Kissinger's efforts to achieve détente with the Soviet Union, China's number-one enemy at that moment.

"The Soviet Union," railed Deng, "is the country which most zealously preaches peace and is the most dangerous source of war." Quite a change of attitude, it seemed, since the civil war days, when Mao sought advice from the Kremlin. The tension in the Great Hall finally eased when the People's Liberation Army band broke into "The Yellow Rose of Texas."

During the three-year interval since my visit with Princess Ida, it was obvious that bits and pieces of Western technology had come to Beijing. The biggest crowd-stopper in town was the new foot-activated front door of the Beijing Hotel, which magically slid open and closed as each guest entered. Orange-and-blue motorized street sweepers had replaced the old women broom brigades. Electric hair dryers and other modern home appliances were on display in the windows of the *Qianmen* (Front Gate) and *Wanfujin* (Well of the Emperor's Mansion) department stores, while the "Day and Night Grocery Store" offered frozen TV dinners.

Local residents were also being introduced to American sports. Men's basketball practice had replaced mass military drills in Tiananmen Square—at least while we were there. Today, basketball is a major sport in China, having produced Yao Ming, the seven-foot giant of the Houston Rockets.

It wasn't until after his defeat by Jimmy Carter that Ford told me about his conversation with Mao. We were flying around the U.S. together in a private plane. The former president was giving a series of political science lectures to college students that I was covering for an article in *Fortune*. He mentioned how surprised he was by the doddering old chairman's grasp of world affairs. But, he said, the translation process from Mao's stuttering Hunanese into Mandarin, and finally into English, was painful. "It was as if the Communist leader had lost control of his tongue," Ford recalled.

Part of the time, he said, Mao's two interpreters had to rely on lip reading. When that failed, Ford described how the chairman, who died the following year, had gripped a soft lead pencil with his shaky right hand and scribbled a few characters. In spite of these communication difficulties,, Mao made clear his displeasure with what he characterized as Ford's "futile arms negotiations" with Soviet President Leonid Brezhnev. But there was no question in Ford's mind that Mao's head was still clear. So much for the claim made by several China experts at the time of the meeting that the Great Helmsman was "gaga."

While in Beijing with Ford, I repeated my request to revisit Henan. "You must write to the Foreign Affairs Ministry," came the broken-record reply, and for the next six years I fired off periodic letters and telegrams that were never answered. Then, unexpectedly, in 1981 an invitation came. By that time, I had become a senior writer for *Fortune,* which was interested in China's "creeping capitalism," as the magazine referred to the country's entrepreneurial reawakening.

For two weeks in a Toyota van, rented with a driver from the Tourist Auto Car Brigade and a guide borrowed from the All-China Journalists Association, my wife Helen, and I zipped down Henan's new, poplar-lined ribbons of blacktop. Following behind in a jeep was a medical doctor in the event we became ill.

The formerly barren, silt-covered Central Plain was green with wheat, corn, sorghum, soybeans, tobacco, and cotton. The ancient towns and villages to which I had delivered relief supplies in 1947 still stood. But, stripped of their ancient protective walls, and stretched helter-skelter to accommodate new schools, factories, and workers' apartments, they now encroached on the surrounding farmland.

Most surprising of all were Kaifeng's sidewalks, strewn with fresh vegetables sold by people who pocketed the proceeds. Managers of the cigarette factories in Xuchang were also being measured by profits, as well as production, and were offering bonuses called "award pay" to the best workers. A few years earlier, those practices would have been branded "unrepentant capitalist backsliding." Everywhere, it seemed, the Marxian dictum "From each according to his abilities, to each according to his needs," was being replaced by the capitalist idea "More pay for more work." But then, as blunt-speaking Deng Xiaoping once said, "Capitalism is better than feudalism."

Arriving at each town, I was surprised—and not a little embarrassed—by the huge crowds lined up five or ten deep along the road, all applauding our arrival on cue. I had brought along more than a hundred photographs taken of these same places thirty-four years earlier. But not one person admitted recognizing anyone in the old pictures. And nobody recalled ever seeing me before, although no other American had ever visited some of those remote villages. The people, it was clear, still feared being punished by the Communist authorities for having once associated with a "foreign devil."

The centerpiece of Henan's development, we found, was the 350-foot-high, 1,000-foot-long Yellow River dam, erected at the foreboding "Gate of Three Demons" (*Sanmenxia*) Gorge at the western edge of the province. In 1957, 100,000 Chinese laborers, supervised by Soviet engineers, had started its construction. But from then on the project languished, stricken by technical and political setbacks.

Before the dam was half-built, the blueprints had to be sent back to St. Petersburg for drastic changes because the Russians had never encountered a river with so much sediment. That problem was solved, but in 1960 all the Soviet experts were expelled as relations between the two countries deteriorated. Then the building of the power plant inside the dam got bogged down in the Cultural Revolution. Finally, in 1973, the combined power and flood-control project was competed, turning what had been "China's Sorrow" into the country's biggest irrigation ditch.

Today, Henan faces a new kind of sorrow—an AIDS epidemic almost as out of control as was the once-rampantly surging Yellow River. The epidemic began in 1999, when, to cope with a blood plasma shortage, local companies and hospitals started offering donors the equivalent of $5 U.S. a pint. Poor peasants leapt at the opportunity to make some easy money. Most of them had never heard of AIDS. Nor did they realize their blood was being pooled, so that any contaminated contributions would infect a whole batch. After the plasma was extracted, the residue, consisting mostly of red cells, was reinjected into the donors, further spreading the disease.

At first, local authorities tried to hide the fact that more than one million people in Henan had become HIV positive. Then, making matters worse, AIDS victims demanding medical assistance were beaten up or jailed by the local authorities. One of the most violent mass protests occurred in Weishi, a former stopover for my truck convoys. Only belatedly were members of the World Health Organization allowed in to help, as they finally were during the subsequent SARS epidemic.

In 1989, as the fortieth anniversary of the fall of Shanghai and the end of the Revolution approached, *Life* decided to send me back there again to write a commemorative article. The CBS "Sunday Morning" TV show, hosted by Charles Kuralt, also asked to cover my return as part of a ninety-minute special on China. What caught the interest of both the magazine and the network was another revolution that seemed to be simmering in Shanghai—this one sparked by Chinese students, regarded as firebrands in their country's growing outcry for democracy.

Landing there in April, I was amazed how outspoken the once docile students had become. Obedience had always been the pillar of their upbringing. But that obviously was no longer so. At Fudan University, Shanghai's Harvard, some five hundred students in its Center for American Studies were being taught how democracy and a free economy were supposed to work. They were mad because it wasn't working in China, and they were willing to tell that to anyone who would listen. It was also evident that American magazines, movies, music, and TV were further stirring their yearnings for reform. "Here in China," they groused, "the more knowledgeable you are, the less money you earn." They blamed that on a carryover from the Cultural Revolution, that equated education with incompetence.

By late May, thousands of students were massing every day in the People's Park, where the racecourse used to be, demanding more opportunity and more freedom. But in Shanghai, government officials wisely resisted calling in the tanks to fire on the student demonstrators as the authorities in Beijing did in Tiananmen Square.

It wasn't just the students in Shanghai who were seething. Although urban planners there had set their sights on a greatly expanded international airport, an updated telephone system, and the city's first subway, there was also unrest in the business community. Local managers complained that the central government was siphoning off too much of the city's profits. "We feed the cow in Shanghai, and they milk it in Beijing," an English-speaking executive told me.

Before leaving Shanghai, I decided to stop in at the decaying building on the Bund formerly occupied by our Time–Life bureau. It currently belonged to the Harbor Navigation Administration. My interpreter explained to two young clerks poring over a pile of papers up on the third floor that it was there in that same office where I had written my final dispatches as the Communists marched in. They looked up in disbelief. "This only happens in the movies," one of them exclaimed.

I felt fortunate in being able to cover Shanghai's development during several more visits prior to the historic day in 1997 when China retook possession of Hong Kong. Shanghai and the British Crown Colony had always suffered a strange love-hate relationship—not quite competitors, but certainly not friends. In 1949, when I moved the Time–Life bureau to Hong Kong, it was still a haven for British colonials who wanted the good life without working too hard. What made it such a magnet for foreign companies after that was not just its deep, protected anchorage, high hills, and spacious views, but the laissez-faire attitude of its British-run government. Yet, it could never match the excitement of Shanghai.

In 1997, as Britain's lease on Hong Kong was about to expire and the two cities were preparing to be wed under the flag of the People's Republic, *Fortune* sent me back to both places to cover their marriage. The two metropolises, I reported, had in effect traded places. Hong Kong's thriving capitalist economy had become the eighth largest in the world. Real estate prices had shot up so preposterously high that many office buildings put up in the seventies were being torn down and replaced by soaring steel-and-glass towers. Nothing seemed rooted in Hong Kong but the pursuit of money.

Watching Hong Kong celebrate the "handover," as the transfer of its sovereignty to China was called, I was struck by the sharp contrast between that peaceful event and the convulsions Shanghai went through as the Communists were about to take control in 1949. I couldn't help but recall those terror-filled last days, when suspected Communist agents were given drumhead trials before being dumped in the street and shot point-blank through the head.

The midnight ceremony in Hong Kong was lit by dazzling fireworks and covered by a foreign media invasion, some six thousand strong. The pipes and drums of the Black Watch were joined by the band of the Scots Guards, the Highland Band and the Gurkha Band in a final symbolic gesture. I watched Prince Charles in effect give the bride away, then, together with her last British guardian, Governor Chris Patten, board the royal yacht *Britannia* and sail out of Hong Kong harbor. This extravaganza, treated like a glittering Hollywood spectacular, was beamed by satellite to the four corners of the earth.

At the same time, I found that Shanghai, although still recovering from almost half a century of Communist neglect, was furiously building more brawn, threatening to become an economic powerhouse again—and perhaps pull past its old rival. Once again, landing in that seething metropolis was like jumping into a cauldron. The city's nonstop assault on the senses was caused not only by the impatient honking of a thousand taxis gridlocked on Nanjing Road or the deafening tattoo of jackhammers biting into bedrock or the new crop of singsong girls populating hundreds of karaoke bars. It was also caused by the capitalistic fever gripping practically everyone of its fourteen million citizens.

Most surprising to me was the garden of gleaming new glass-and-concrete office towers popping up out of the mud flats of Pudong across the Huangpu River from the Bund and the old business district. Shanghai had yet to fill many of those skyscraper shells, though the occupancy rate was rapidly rising from the paltry fifteen percent when they first opened. A network of new subways, speedways, tunnels, and bridges linked the city's districts.

But whether or not Shanghai ever supplants Hong Kong as the financial engine driving China, its residents were already on a spending spree. Many slum dwellers without water or electricity had cell phones. Appliance stores were bursting with VCRs, CD players, and camcorders. "We were too conservative. We had no idea we would be so popular and making so much money," confided Domenico De Sole, Gucci's CEO, when he opened Shanghai's first foreign haute couture store. Watching the svelte Chinese models show off Gucci's wares, I was reminded of how Mao Zedong's Great Leap Forward dismally failed, while Deng Xiaoping's leap into "market socialism" hurtled ahead practically out of control, as the annual rise in the country's GDP (Gross Domestic Product) exceeded eight percent and its international trade surplus mounted with staggering speed.

The success of China's burgeoning capitalism was certainly understandable. Its people always were entrepreneurial, a trait not even Mao could erase. I remember Stalin once complained that the East Germans didn't cotton well to Communism. "It fits them like a saddle fits a cow," he remarked. The same, I sensed, was true of the Chinese. In the old days, even the lowliest Shanghai shopkeepers loved to bargain with their customers. In many stores there was a special "morning price" to get business rolling. Or, if you shook your head and walked away, the shopkeeper would come running down the street in hot pursuit offering a sizable discount. It was clear nobody in China liked losing a sale.

Before leaving Shanghai on that visit in 1997, I decided to retrace my former morning walk from the Correspondents' Club in Broadway Mansions (renamed the Shanghai Mansion Hotel), to the building on the Bund formerly occupied by the Time–Life office. The wide waterfront promenade now pulsated with exercisers, sword dancers, slow-motion shadow boxers practicing the ancient art of tai chi chuan, joggers, tumblers, wrestlers, even ballroom dancers learning a few basic steps. Old women fox-trotted together, and so did old men. But as I watched those gyrating figures I could still see ghost images of the blind and crippled beggars sprawled on that pavement with their hands outstretched for alms.

By the fiftieth anniversary of the People's Republic in 1999, I had already seen how Beijing and the cities of coastal China had been transformed under Deng Xiaoping's and Jiang Zemin's economic reforms. But what had happened to the four former Nationalist strongholds—Shenyang, Taiyuan, Xuzhou, and Nanjing, where the crucial battles of the civil war had been fought? Were they stuck in a time warp? Or were they also leapfrogging into the twenty-first century? Before ending my long association with China, I felt a compelling urge to find out.

Fortune, once again, was delighted to send me back. This time it didn't take years of cajoling cables and letters to wring an invitation from the foreign ministry. Accompanied by my wife Helen and photographer Fritz Hoffmann, we began the return trek in Shenyang, or Mukden, as the former capital of Manchuria was called. The ghost city of one million destitute residents that was being overrun by Communist General Lin Biao's soldiers when I hurriedly left had swelled to a population of 6.8 million. New skyscrapers were sprouting everywhere. But a few of the old landmarks remained. The one hundred-foot-high Soviet victory obelisk topped with a Russian tank still guarded the railroad station jammed in 1948 with soldiers and civilians selling their belongings to buy a rail ticket to safety. It didn't look that different. A number of the city's 400,000 unemployed workers were selling their TVs and radios there to eke out money for food.

Other residents, however, had become affluent and were not averse to being seen in skin-tight Ralph Lauren jeans or wearing flashy Gucci ties. The Tschurin Company department store had survived, but that drab Soviet temple of commerce was now a glitzy Chinese emporium filled with jewelry and watches. Everywhere, the once-deserted, windswept thoroughfares were locked in a honking mishmash of bikes, buses, and taxis, except for those streets being torn up by ubiquitous work gangs of orange-jacketed jailbirds. Obviously, the corruption that had plagued Chiang's regime in Shenyang was still a problem under the Communists. We'd just arrived when it was reported that First Deputy Mayor Ma Xiangdong and two other senior city officials had been arrested for gambling away $3 million of public funds in a Macao casino.

After the civil war, Shenyang had become a center of state-run heavy industry. The city continued to rely on its smoke-belching old smelters, and the air was heavy with smog. But it was already replacing them with pristine, high-tech plants, including those belonging to IBM and Hewlett-Packard. But they, too, were causing a problem. While the new, mostly foreign-financed plants (ironically, some backed by Taiwan firms) were cleaner, more efficient, and more profitable, they didn't employ nearly as many people. And the frequent street protests among the jobless were not always peaceful. State employment agencies offered retraining classes, while the Workers' Cultural Palace provided such diversions as disco dancing—would you believe—starting at dawn.

More surprising than the influx of big U.S. corporations was the number of pioneering Americans settling in this freezing, far-north metropolis, visited only by a few foreign fur traders in the 1940s. The U.S. entrepreneurs were a diverse crowd. Tom Kirkwood, president of the Shenyang Shawnee (he came from Shawnee, Pennsylvania) Candy Company, proved to be a whirlwind manufacturer and promoter of a chewy TootsieRoll-type candy called Longhorn Bars that he sold in Shenyang by the truckload. "My marketing plan was simple," he said. "Chinese children love candy and cowboys."

One of the most successful American-run ventures was a chain of English-language schools for four-year-olds and up. "Chinese parents are determined to see their kids get ahead," said Christopher Williams, the school's founder. "They think English is the key." His business was booming with 2,500 students and 72 American, Canadian and Chinese teachers spread over five schools.

Williams' schools had to shut down for a week after the U.S mistakenly bombed the Chinese embassy in Belgrade. But his business suffered no damage. The American consulate was not so fortunate. Organized mobs smashed every window, forcing the staff to take refuge in a hotel. Still that was nothing compared to the wrath experienced by Consul General Angus Ward and his staff after the Communists captured the city in 1948.

The compulsion of Chinese parents to teach their children English was also evident in Taiyuan. When we first entered the shiny new Shanxi Grand Hotel lobby, a young crew-cut boy stopped me. "My name is Simon," he said. "I'm eight years old." Then he handed me his printed calling card, which included his own e-mail address.

What a difference half a century makes! When I left Marshal Yan Xishan's old walled capital, children were starving, not chatting up foreigners. The hills around the city, once honeycombed with Communist gun emplacements, were now being mined for coal, iron ore, and gypsum. A children's playground with brightly painted swings and slides had replaced the old dirt airstrip that kept the city alive during the airlift. In fact, it was hard to find anything left from the civil war days except for the massive North Gate of the old city wall through which Mao's troops poured. It was being preserved as a Communist victory monument.

Unlike Shenyang, which embraced economic reform at an early stage, Taiyuan had been slow in moving towards capitalism. In some ways this was a blessing. With its new broad, tree-lined boulevards, the city was very inviting. But here, too, the Communist legacy was being slowly dismantled. Marshal Yan's huge arsenal, first converted into a plant belonging to the Taiyuan Heavy Machinery Group, became a classic example of an overstaffed, inefficient state-owned enterprise. Reorganized and slimmed down, the company, now known as TZ, makes everything from giant cranes that were used for building the Yangtze River dams to satellite-launching towers (which we were not permitted to see).

"Until 1997 everything was government-planned," said TZ's vice general manager, Tang Bao Ren. "But the company has since been decentralized and the number of workers reduced." Then, realizing he was talking to the representative of a capitalist magazine, he added brightly, "Today our workers can buy TZ shares on the Shanghai stock exchange."

Few foreigners live in this sweltering, bustling interior city of three million. Even so, TZ managed to establish eleven joint ventures, three of them with American companies. A shiny new twenty-five million, joint-venture

Coca Cola bottling plant has also sprouted in Taiyuan, turning out 400,000 cases of the soft drink a month. But you had to wonder if the city's fathers quite got the hang of this capitalist thing. Smiling portraits of officially designated "model workers" lined the main thoroughfare, still named Welcome Chairman Mao Street. And, while corruption may not have been as flagrant as it was in Shenyang, a scam in Taiyuan involving government bureaucrats caught transferring municipal funds into their own accounts made the front page of the *Wall Street Journal*. But, then, as the newspaper pointed out, bank fraud is a countrywide affliction in China, with eight thousand cases, totaling more than twelve billion, having been apprehended in the year 2000 alone.

On our last night in Taiyuan, we were invited to a banquet given by the deputy mayor, who could press the flesh and slap a back as well as any American politician. He failed to show up. Later, we discovered he'd been suddenly summoned to Beijing, not for fraud, but for his laxness in dealing with the outlawed Falun Gong, a spiritual movement that blended exercise with meditation. In Beijing, a couple of Falun Gong members have since set themselves afire to protest the harsh government crackdown there. But, apparently, in Taiyuan they'd been allowed to openly practice their quasi-religion, which the Communist leaders in Beijing considered a threat to their authority. Rest assured, we didn't mind missing yet another one of those sumptuous meals featuring such regional specialties as fried cicadas and stewed snake, followed by a tortoise with the shell still on—that last delicacy served only to the guest of honor.

Thinking about the government ban of the Falun Gong, I recalled how Marshal Yan Xishan had established a Heart Cleansing Institute in Taiyuan to purify the thoughts of his subjects. The objectives of the Falun Gong movement didn't seem so different. They both encouraged prayers and meditation, which the old Marshal used to practice at the city's main temple, named the Monastery of Endless Happiness.

When Birns and I left Taiyuan in 1948, running and ducking to reach the airstrip during a deafening mortar attack, I remember glancing back at the twin pagodas of that Buddhist monastery and thinking what a ridiculous name for a place of worship in a war-torn city being put through such torture. When we flew out of Taiyuan on this trip, I gazed down at the shiny twin towers of the new forty-two-story Shanxi International Trade Center, which dominated the skyline the way the twin towers of the Pagoda of Endless Happiness used to. Yes, I thought, this soaring steel-and-glass edifice symbolizes Taiyuan's new capitalist religion.

Xuzhou, the city associated with the great Battle of the Huai-Hai, was not as modern as Shenyang or Taiyuan. Most of its older buildings had survived, making it more resonant of the China I used to know. It hadn't even inaugurated regular air service. Yet it was a far different place than the panicked city of 250,000 that I left in 1948. Nationalist officers were sweeping up civilians from the refugee-packed streets to dig trenches and patch the city's protective wall. Trucks, mule carts, and rickshaws filled with wounded soldiers struggled in from the battlefield, twenty-five miles to the east.

City officials now were making big plans for their citizens, speaking grandly of a "Euro-Asia land bridge," a proposed highway stretching from Xuzhou through Siberia to Amsterdam. Giving the city its biggest economic boost was the Jin Shan Qiao (Golden Garden Bridge) Development Zone. In it were Japanese, German, and American factories. An entire village, Long Tan Gardens, had been built for foreign executives, resembling a new housing development in Anywhere, U.S.A. The city's new supermarkets, air-conditioned just short of frostbite, bulged with packaged fruits, vegetables, and meats, some from as far away as New Zealand. And we witnessed a fifteen-minute wait for a seat in the Kentucky Fried Chicken franchise, which had a lifesize, welcoming statue of Colonel Sanders standing out front.

But Xuzhou also retained a keen sense of its past. We were shown a recently completed sleek, modern museum of Han dynasty art. (Xuzhou was the home town of Liu Bang, the first Han Dynasty emperor, circa 206 B.C.) Another, older museum containing Battle of the Huai-Hai memorabilia attracted 600,000 Chinese visitors a year. "Huai-Hai was like your Gettysburg," the curator explained, repeating the comparison that Mao's generals had made during the war. I was fascinated by this museum's three-dimensional maps, dioramas, film clips, and photographs, showing the Communist side of this epic battle, in which more than a million men faced each other at close range. When I showed the curator some of *Life*'s photographs taken from the Nationalist side, he insisted on having them copied for the museum.

What I wanted to do most was find the little village of Zhouzhuang. It was from a nearby hilltop that Birns and I had observed the fierce Nationalist attack and Communist counter-attack that proved to be the climactic battle of the war. Still etched in my memory was the sleepless night we spent there, in a mud hut, listening to artillery shells scream overhead while the pounding pulse from my oncoming bout of typhoid beat in my ears. It was a terrible dilemma. Though I desperately wanted to cover that million-man battle to its bitter end, my fever and throbbing head told me to hurry back to Shanghai.

On my return visit to the battleground, I discovered there were three villages named Zhouzhuang, all within thirty miles of each another. Bumping over pitted dirt roads, we naturally went to the two wrong ones first. Finally, at the foot of Dragon Hill, some twenty-five miles east of Xuzhou, we found the Zhouzhuang where I'd spent that terrifying night.

Compared with the transformation of Xuzhou, little seemed changed in this poor village. Ducks, chickens, pigs, and bare-bottomed children scampered through the muddy streets lined with thatched-roofed dwellings. During the war, the place had been ringed with tanks, trenches, and mud pillboxes, and was almost deserted. Now, at least the place was at peace. I showed some of the wartime photographs to a few of the oldsters who had lived through the battle. "That's my grandmother," shouted one, pointing to the picture of an old woman defiantly standing her ground amidst the machine gun positions outside her mud house.

I climbed the rocky hill where Jack Birns and I had encountered General Li Mi, commander of the Nationalist Thirteenth Army Group, directing artillery fire. About a hundred soldiers had been sprawled over the craggy slope, weapons in their laps, eating their evening bowls of rice. Now, quarry workers were turning this hill into gravel. In a year or two, I realized, the hill would no longer exist, the gravel having all been used to build more sky-scrapers in Xuzhou.

Reaching the top, I remembered watching the battle progress as the sun dipped below the horizon and General Li shouted curt commands into a field phone. Ahead of the artillery, tracers from the 37mm guns on Li's tanks had cut red streaks through the blackness. Occasional flares lit the sky. It was all still so clear in my mind. My reverie was abruptly broken when the quarry workers set off a succession of dynamite blasts, a deafening reminder of what China's civil war sounded like.

There were few sounds of battle by which to remember the fall of Nanjing. Only the panicked cries and curses of people trying to escape from the Nationalist capital. Well, some things haven't changed. Boarding a train in Nanjing, the wild shoving and pushing was almost as bad as it was in April 1949. But Nanjing now had more than five million people, four times its wartime population. Even so, it had become one of the most livable cities in China, with many parks, tree-shaded streets, and terraced apartments. It was also booming. Jin Zhong Qing, the vice governor of Jiangsu Province bragged to us at yet another one of those sumptuous banquets that Nanjing had already attracted 125 *Fortune* 500 companies, and would soon be adding more.

Vast quantities of goods were now moving in and out of the same Yangtze River docks where American and British warships were formerly tied up. Yu Yong Je, the deputy office manager of the Panda Electronics Group, who wasn't even born then, nevertheless described how his company had all of its factory equipment down on the dock ready to be shipped to Taiwan when the Communists entered the city. "But the workers refused to go," he said. "So here we are, still in Nanjing."

The river traffic had become so heavy that many of the ships were being turned around in a day. "You get unloaded too quick to have any fun," complained Constance Xyristakis, chief engineer of the Greek freighter *Aris,* perhaps referring to the seedy massage parlors that hired a number of the women laid off by the state-owned factories. "There's always another ship waiting for your berth."

Nanjing was not on the conventional tourist route but busloads of children came from all over China to climb the three hundred gleaming white stone steps up Purple Mountain. At the top, they gazed at the crypt holding the remains of Sun Yat-sen, the man who overthrew the Manchu dynasty and founded the Republic of China. It was ironic, or so it seemed to me, that both Taiwan, whose formal name is the Republic of China, and the mainland, which is the People's Republic of China, today lay claim to Sun's legacy.

My most vivid memories of Nanjing, the ones that followed me there in the year 2000, were of the day before the city changed hands. I remembered the arm-waving moneychangers still plying their trade at Sun Yat-sen Circle, perhaps to stifle their fear of what lies ahead. Now, young lovers snuggled together there at night, trying to figure out their future. And then there was the ridiculous sight of salvage crews at Ming Palace Airport, which were continuing to turn the wings of Nationalist air force planes into pots and pans. Or were they, too, merely working hard to blot out the danger of that day, the same way we war correspondents counted on the excitement of covering a battle to dissipate our fears? The former airport was now the site of the Jincheng motorcycle factory, where we watched a fast-moving, dust-free assembly line churn out engines for Japanese Suzukis at the rate of one every two minutes.

Nor would I ever forget that last evening in Nanjing as the city lay ominously quiet after being swept by a wave of looting. Photographer Carl Mydans and I didn't know what to expect. We were catnapping, trying to get a little sleep before the attack began. The defending artillery batteries fired a few perfunctory shots, that was all, before we heard the sound of distant bugles announcing the Communists' arrival. The Nationalist capital, I then realized, belonged to Mao Zedong, as the rest of China soon would.

In the years ahead, I know the sights, the sounds, and the smells of China will continue to be a part of my being, just as they have been for the past fifty-eight years. Simply reading the word "China" in a newspaper or magazine summons vivid memories that don't seem to dim. Clearly as ever, I can hear the cacophony of Shanghai. I can still see the yellow, loess-covered Central Plain, interspersed with mud villages where the Nationalist and

Communist soldiers and militiamen played cat and mouse as a prelude to their all-out civil war. And I'll never forget the view from the air of those two mighty rivers, the Yellow and the Yangtze, slithering down from misty purple peaks and snaking across the entire country to the sea.

But even better than the land, I still see the weathered faces laughing at the slightest humorous provocation, or crying out in pain for a lack of food, or for the loss of a son or daughter killed in the fighting. Clearest of all, I remember men and women substituting for beasts of burden: pulling plows, pushing irrigation pumps, and struggling with heavy millstones to grind their wheat. And I'm stunned at how most of that primitive, four-thousand-year-old hand work gave way to modern production in just my lifetime.

When I think of the two warring political figures, Mao and Chiang, and how the United States refrained from getting drawn into their great battle, I'm surprised how that lesson was lost on us when the same kind of civil strife broke out in Vietnam. I don't know of one foreign correspondent that covered China's civil war who would have recommended our getting into that morass, trying to "win the hearts and minds" of Ho Chi Minh's countrymen—a miscalculation that cost 58,000 American lives. As a journalist, however, I willingly covered that war on and off during the sixties and seventies, before being evacuated on one of the last helicopters out of Saigon.

Most surprising of all when I think of China today as it gains superpower status, is the waning culture clash between East and West that used to be so striking. The mandarin executive has shed his long blue gown and wears a suit and tie just like his American counterpart, although some still favor the clicking beads of the age-old abacus over an electronic calculator. But he spouts the same business jargon as he wheels and deals to flood the planet with his "made in China" products. Even the courteous Shanghai taxi driver has become as caustic as any New York City cabbie. And in the newly air-conditioned food markets, the chirp of caged crickets is now drowned out by chirping cell phones. But the frozen dumplings available there can't compare with the captivating aroma and flavor of those formerly steamed in big brass kettles and hawked on the street.

This cultural exchange hasn't been all West to East. San Francisco is where, according to my taste, you'll find the finest Chinese cooking—and even see a few tourists sporting around town in pedicabs. You can also watch giant pandas at play in the National Zoo in Washington and view the Great Wall in Disney World. Not surprisingly, the Rock and Roll Hall of Fame, a bastion of American culture, picked the imaginative Chinese-born architect I. M. Pei to design its building in Cleveland. The dragon that symbolized the China that I chased as a foreign correspondent is clearly breathing new fire all around the world. Yet, it's the historic Middle Kingdom, as the vast country was once called, that has forever left its mark on me.

Writing this book has been an exciting journey back to the beginning of my career as a journalist. I am deeply grateful for the cheerful support of my wife Helen, who never complained about the long hours I spent poring over old notes and secluded with my word processor, instead of being with her. I would also like to thank William P. Gray. He not only rescued me, a frustrated relief worker and aspiring journalist in China, and recommended me for a job with Time Inc., but also introduced me to Helen before he died.

I am also grateful to my former comrade-in-arms, photographer Jack Birns, for the exciting times we spent together covering the China civil war battles in 1948 and 1949. *Life* picture editor, Barbara Baker Burrows, was very helpful in finding a number of Jack's photographs taken while he was on the staff, and in granting reprint rights to use them.

Jay McCullough, my editor at the Lyons Press, deserves credit for suggesting that I write this as a memoir, and for giving me good guidance along the way. Mildred Gokey Brucker refreshed my memory about events in the early chapters. Also, my agent Carol Mann lent her helpful support, as she has for so many years.

Several books provided useful background information: *The Good Earth*, by Pearl Buck; *Red Star Over China*, by Edgar Snow; *Personal History*, by

Vincent Sheean; *Thunder Out of China*, by Theodore H. White and Annalee Jacoby; *Stilwell and the American Experience in China, 1911-1945*, by Barbara Tuchman; *China Hands*, by Peter Rand; *Harry & Teddy*, by Thomas Griffith; *The Soong Dynasty*, by Sterling Seagrave; *Decisive Encounters*, by Odd Arne Westad; *China Pilot*, by Felix Smith; *Covering China*, by John Roderick; and *Shanghai*, by Stella Dong.

Finally, I would like to thank Henry Luce, whom we affectionately called, "the proprietor," and the other editors at *Time*, *Life*, and *Fortune*, for sending me on the odysseys that became the fodder for this book.

—ROY ROWAN
GREENWICH, CT
APRIL, 2004

Churchill, Winston, 62

CIA. *See* External Survey Department

CLARA (Communist Liberated Area Relief Association), 65, 66–67

Cleveland, Harlan, 38, 59, 68–70, 84, 89

Clothing, relief, 22–23, 72–73

Coalition government, 63, 75–76

Communist Manifesto (Marx), 198

Communists. *See also* Mao Zedong

after the revolution, 219–21

attack on *Amethyst,* 194–98

attack on Nanjing, 190–91

attack on Taiyuan, 126, 131–32

attack on Weifang, 97–98

attacks in Henan, 28, 44, 48

attacks on railways, 32, 77

Battle of the Huai-Hai, 145–59

birthplace of party, 19–20, 198

capture of General Hao, 67–68

capture of Mukden, 107–19

capture of Shanghai, 213–18

capture of Zhengzhou, 86

CLARA (Communist Liberated Area Relief Association), 65, 66–67

crossing the Yangtze, 187–88

in Fukou, 55–56

infiltrating CNRRA, 58

Long March, 66

maneuvering by, 99–100

and relief supplies, 47, 64–65, 66–67, 72

and smuggled contraband, 38

surrender of Beijing to, 141–44

Confucius, 124

Conrad, Joseph, 7

Consort (ship), 196

Convoys, relief. *See also* Railways, 43–59

in Flooded Area, 53, 54–55

flying supplies to, 44–45

harassment of, 46, 71

Kaifeng to Xihua, 47–58, 71–73

Wunudian to Yanling, 51–53

Corruption, 21, 29–30, 32, 72–73

Coward, Noel, 37

Crouch, Sue, 213

Cruel Separation (Lobo), 171, 173

Cultural exchange, East/West, 243–44

Cultural Revolution, 220, 231

Currency

Chiang's reforms, 163–68

devaluation of, 163

D

Dahu (wealthy families), 164

Dalaohu ("big tigers"), 166

Danger, addiction to, 121–22